JOHN MORDAUNT

12/20

FACING UP TO AIDS

JOHN MORDAUNT

FACING UP TO AIDS

As told to
John Masterson

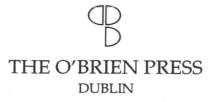

THE O'BRIEN PRESS
DUBLIN

First Published 1989 by The O'Brien Press Ltd.,
20 Victoria Road, Rathgar, Dublin 6, Ireland.

British Library Cataloguing in Publication Data
Mordaunt, John
Facing up to Aids: a story of courage and hope.
1. Aids (Disease) Psychological aspects
I. Title II. Masterson, John
362.1'969792
ISBN 0-86278-182-5 (hardback)
0-86278-191-4 (paperback)
10 9 8 7 6 5 4 3 2 1

Cover Design: The Graphiconies
Typeset at The O'Brien Press
Printed by Leinster Leader Naas

Introduction

John Mordaunt moved to London from Dublin in the summer of 1987. He lives in a North London house divided into four well-equipped self-contained flats. It is in Tottenham, an area becoming fashionable. It is comfortable and expensive, compared to the lot of many young London immigrants. There is a flash-looking telephone on the floor. He has a video and a colour TV.

The links with Ireland are evident. His flatmate, a friend for over ten years, has a strong Dublin accent. The tapes he has been playing are Clannad and U2. There is a framed photograph of his mother and sister Avril on the shelf. And a photograph of his brother Niall receiving a special achievement award for a story he entered in a competition. Niall is thirteen and is confined to a wheelchair.

Twice a week John has his flat cleaned, clothes washed and ironed and gets help with the weekly shopping. His diary is full. The phone rings regularly asking him to fulfil speaking engagements. It frequently rings with people asking for advice. Occasionally there is a request for a television interview.

John Mordaunt has AIDS. He is twenty-nine years old and has been a heroin addict for about half of his life. He has not "used" since May 1987 but still takes his abstinence one day at a time and is on a Methadone maintenance programme. The table in his living room is cluttered with half-empty bottles of prescribed pills and every now and again he takes a mouthful of Methadone. He is a walking encyclopaedia on drugs — legal and prescribed — on addicts and addiction, and on HIV infection and the facilities available for people with the virus.

John was told of his diagnosis in January 1986 and almost died at that time. He pulled through, only to attempt suicide twice in the following six months. The first attempt was serious and only pure luck saved him. The second perhaps a bit half-hearted.

Around the middle of 1987, after fourteen years of phenomenal drug abuse, he felt ready to quit heroin and resolved to spend his remaining time doing all he could to prevent the spread of AIDS. For the first time since his childhood in Dublin, life has some meaning other than where to get the next fix.

Chapter 1

FINGLAS - EARLY DAYS

John was born in London in October 1958 and a few months later the family moved back to the close-knit community of Dublin's inner city where his parents Jack and Carmel Mordaunt had grown up. John was their first child and until he was six he lived near his grandparents and relations, surrounded by neighbours whose families often had lived in the same streets for generations. The Mordaunt family lived in what John describes as a tenement in Hogan's Place at the back of Pearse Street. This consisted of public housing, built by Dublin Corporation, and the main characteristic of the area at the time was poverty.

His father was a sailor, often away from home for long periods. When at home he gambled and John's earliest memories are of his mother and father fighting about money and gambling. His father gambles to this day and though it is now more under control it has remained a source of tension in the marriage for the last thirty years. With his father away so much John became close to his mother from an early age.

The family lived in the house in Hogan's Place with John as an only child until he was six years old. Then in 1963 a Corporation house fell down in nearby Fenian Street, killing two children. The residents got together and marched on the Corporation offices. The Corporation accelerated its policy of clearing the inner city and moving the inhabitants out to the belt of new houses being built on the outskirts of Dublin to combat the housing shortage in the city. In 1964 the family moved to Finglas.

Finglas at that time was completely undeveloped and John remembers it as green fields out in the wilds. 'They hadn't even got roads when we arrived. It was dirt tracks. They built the houses and forgot to build the fuckin' roads.'

His mother also hated it. 'Hogan's Place was a tenement. Thousands of families lived in them at the time. I think there were seven houses with fifty-two families in them and we all had one room. John was nearly seven and we were handed the keys of a three-bedroomed house which was a miracle with only one child. We were just told to "git" because the houses were literally falling. So we moved to Finglas in November and I hated it. After being in a close-knit community, near your own father, near Jack's people.'

They knew no one. There were no shops. There was nothing to do. It was a disaster after the intimate environment of Hogan's Place. Both parents hated it. But they were stuck there. They continued to argue, mostly about gambling. John found himself in the middle of nowhere with only his mother and father for company.

'I had some bad problems with wanting to be surrounded by my family, because I had lived in an extended family in Hogan's Place with my granny, aunties, uncles and friends all around, and suddenly to be stuck out in Finglas with just my mother and father was quite strange.'

The arrival within the space of a year of his brother Patrick and sister Avril only made things more difficult. 'Within eleven months I went from being the centre of attention to being relegated to third place and I hated it. When they were young I did some terrible things to the kids ... bouncing them down the stairs and making them eat cigarettes, pouring glue on them - the sort of things that kids do to other kids, you know!' To this day John is happiest when he is the centre of attention.

To make matters worse, his mother suffered from post natal depression. 'I just couldn't cope with being stuck out in a house after being a very free woman with one child and a part-time job. I had always been very active and independent. And then Jack was gambling heavily. Our marriage was a bit rockedy. Gambling is a terrible thing to live with. But we've been together for thirty-one years, so there must be something there.

'Through all this I was at home with the babies and I always talked to John. And if his father didn't come home I'd leave him minding them and I'd go looking for his father in town. Then things would go good for a while and we got a car. Then one Monday we didn't have a car any more. He sold it and put it on a dog. It was a lot of hassle and my depression was getting worse but I never told anybody, only John.

'People would knock at the door from loan companies that I knew nothing about. You'd say to yourself, Oh Jesus, not again. Then Jack got himself very straight.

'But there were always lots of arguments over gambling. It was the one problem. We had a good marriage but for this one fault. And then he'd have a big win and it would be like Christmas. I think John couldn't understand why I would be still nagging. He would be happy when his Daddy was buying him this, that and the other. I knew the following week it would be back to square one.'

John remembers being a chubby intelligent eleven-year-old who felt a bit different from the rest of his mates. He was always fat, and self-conscious about it. But he was also that bit brighter than the rest. He felt unique - he was the one who was going to go that bit further than the rest.

Finglas meanwhile continued to grow. It was a poverty-stricken area and a lot of families living there had social problems of one sort or another. Drugs were a familiar part of the environment. Many of the women, trapped with small children in a new community with a shortage of shops and buses, used Valium.

Even before he was a teenager John remembers thinking about drugs. The sixties came to Ireland late and spilled over into the seventies via the Viet Nam war. This was the first war watched on television and with it came a strong American vibe about alternative ways of living. This appealed to many - with anti-war protests which captured the high moral stance of the time, long hair, friendliness, free and easy attitudes, flamboyant clothes and drugs.

John watched the war on TV and as a twelve-year-old devoured *Newsweek* and *Time* magazines. The way of life portrayed was so different to life in Finglas. It was attractive, and drugs were a part of it.

'I felt bad about my body and I felt fat. But I fitted in. I had some great friends in Finglas, friends who have lasted me all my life, but I remember the first time I ever took drugs, I took some of my mother's Valium. I was about twelve, twelve-and-a-half. I had heard about Valium from some other kids on the street and that if you had some Valium and some cider it was a good hit. So I nicked a few and we bought some cider and we went up the fields, four of us and we took the Valium and drank the cider and we got wrecked. We were twelve-year-old kids stumbling around a field in Finglas chasing cows - out of our minds. It felt natural. It was what everybody was doing. It didn't seem in any way strange. That's one thing that always strikes me about those early years. It didn't strike me that I was doing anything strange. All the people I knew except for those that were still playing football or going to youth clubs were all out playing kiss-chasing and trying to get stoned.

'You have to understand that I lived in an area where in a lot of houses the father was either a gambler or a wife-beater or an alcoholic. Many women were on tranquilisers of one description or another. They got so many from the doctors that most of them never even noticed they were being stolen.'

But if Valium and cider were a hit, the first drugs John remembers with real affection were 'pondies'. Pondrax was a widely available slimming tablet comprised mainly of amphetamines, or 'speed'.

'You'd eat handfuls of them. You could buy them in the chemist. You'd get a girl to go in and buy them because they wouldn't sell them to us because we were so young. Pondrax were brilliant because they gave you energy. You suddenly felt like Superman. You could run and jump and you wanted to go disco boogieing.'

John was in first year in the Patrician Brothers secondary school, doing well, and enjoying himself with

Valium and speed. He wasn't interested in alcohol. The only use he had for cider was to boost the hit from pills.

Chapter 2

HIPPIE LIFE - SOFT DRUGS IN SANTRY

John was an intelligent child and did well in the entrance exam for the Patrician Brothers secondary school. He secured a place in Form 1A, the top stream. In school the intelligence that got him into 1A was also to prove his undoing. He found school easy, very easy. Homework was never a problem. He could do it in class or during breaks. He never needed to take it home. Outside school hours he was totally free to develop his other interests, including drugs. He was a clever, fattish, popular youngster who felt that bit different from the rest.

John went from 1A to 2A and when he was thirteen he first came across 'hash and grass', as cannabis and marijuana were usually known. 'How that happened was I had begun dressing like a hippie - flared jeans, waistcoats, crioses and long hair and I bumped into this other guy who looked like me. He was about sixteen and he became a very good friend of mine. Now he grew his own grass and he invited me down to his house. He had his own bedroom with a stereo in it, big cushions up against the walls, soft lights - and I went into his room and he rolled a big joint of grass. I'd never started smoking cigarettes, for some unknown reason, so my first smoke of anything was a joint of pure grass. I smoked it, and man I felt so relaxed. All the tension seemed to drain out of my body.

'This wasn't Finglas. It was Santry, and Santry was posh. Finglas was the dregs. These people from Santry were really nice and they accepted me as I was and we shared the same interests. We wanted to stop the Viet Nam war. We wanted to get stoned. We were into peace and love. I began going down there quite a lot and I stopped taking Valium and Pondrax and got totally into grass and hash.'

Then one day one of the group had some LSD, or acid as it was universally known. John knew what acid was because books like Timothy Leary's *The Politics of Experience* were required reading for the group and were discussed endlessly. Leary, a Harvard academic who was fired for advocating the use of LSD, advised everyone to 'Turn on, tune in and drop out.' LSD was the answer.

'This was my first tab of acid and I can remember it was like a religious ceremony. It was a big long strip of "window pane" and we had to use a razor blade to cut it up on a mirror. It was LSD in liquidy form held between two pieces of gelatin in cellophane. It was called window pane because that is exactly what it looked like.

'It was handed around like communion. I sat there and I smoked a joint and I remember blowing out the smoke of the joint and it curled into these amazing colours and shapes. It was incredible. Acid opens up a part of your mind that you never even thought about before. It's hard to explain to someone who hasn't done it. You become sensitised. Sex on acid is something else - but that was later.

'The first tab was a profound experience. It was a

14

couple of kids from Santry and Finglas sitting in a darkened room with hippie music playing and blissing out ... that feeling of belonging, not feeling isolated from people any more, a sense of wonder. I mean Finglas was grimy and real and mundane, and acid was the complete opposite. It was spiritual, it was colourful, it held out a promise of something better to come.'

John took LSD as often as he could get it. He began tripping in school where he was still in the A stream.

'I remember a master staring down into my spaced-out eyes saying: "Mordaunt, there is something very strange about you. I can't quite put my finger on it but there is something not right about you." He hadn't a clue that I was sitting there out of my mind on acid. The floor was heaving just like it was breathing, everybody had an aura around them. It was just crazy. I was still thirteen and this was in school. The first time I tripped in school was just before my fourteenth birthday.'

John's leisure time revolved around drugs, his hippie friends and science fiction books and comics. John's London flat is still littered with comics. He has had a lifelong fascination with the artwork and storylines. As a teenager he thought about worlds existing in parallel to ours and thought of drugs as giving a look into these sideways worlds. He began to refer to himself as a 'sideways person', sideways to reality.

'I've often referred to how I felt fundamentally unique. I never felt that anybody else had the depth of feeling that I seemed to have. I would lie in bed and listen to my mother and father screaming at each other and I'd be just crying and feeling ripped to bits ... from the age of about eight to about thirteen every night I'd lie there and I'd lie with my fingers in my ears praying that my mother and father wouldn't start arguing.

'There was only one person I felt I could relate to and that was my friend Ken. I felt my intelligence made me different because I was quite clever. I felt like a stranger in a strange land. Sometimes I felt like these weren't my real parents and this wasn't my real home. It was all a big mistake!

'I felt I should be living in a big huge mansion with everything I wanted instead of a brick shithouse in Finglas! My mother used to say I was a millionaire's bastard!'

Chapter 3

FOURTEEN - THE FIRST FIX

The feeling of being isolated, different and out of place is one that has characterised John's personality throughout his life. It drove him on the one hand to drugs to bring about a feeling of belonging, while on the other hand he liked the feeling of standing out from the crowd, of being a cut above the rest. And it always drove him one step further than the others.

The family wasn't particularly religious. His parents had stopped attending Mass regularly when they moved to Finglas. 'I think my mother decided God had deserted her!' And John's feeling of isolation did not push him in a religious direction.

He wasn't a team person, and while he played some football, he openly admits that the only thing that concerned him was his own performance. Whether the team won or lost was secondary. He was goalkeeper and interested only in how clean a sheet he kept.

And because he was taking drugs and had posh friends in Santry he felt completely alien from the rough environment of Finglas. The locals just didn't seem to be in touch with what he thought was important.

'What I thought was important was loving people, showing affection, being kind - and it wasn't like that in Finglas. It was a tough hard struggle. The typical family was trying to make ends meet. There wasn't a lot of luxury. It was not an environment that was conducive to appreciating the finer things in life. For entertainment there was only one cinema, about a dozen pubs and a few bingo halls.'

Expensive and exotic tastes were way beyond his reach, but from his early teens John was making his own spending money. He remembers lying in bed deciding that he was no longer going to be affected by his parents' arguments. He stopped crying at nights. Instead, from the time he was thirteen, he began to work as a lounge boy in local pubs.

Soon he had enough money to buy his own clothes, sweets and magazines and he also contributed to the family income because there was always a shortage of money. He usually worked two nights during the week and at weekends. A lot of young kids from Finglas had jobs in pubs or supermarkets or shops. They were cheap labour at £1.25 a night. But it wasn't all above board.

'In one of the pubs I was working in I got a great fiddle going with one of the barmen. I was taking home £1.75 a night wages and £30 a night fiddle. The barman used to provide his own spirits and when I would pay for a round of drinks the money for the pints would go into the till but he would pocket the spirits money some of the time. At the end of the night we would split it 60/40 in his favour. I kept trying for 50/50 but never got it!

At the same time all John's values were coming from the States. There was the message that young people could make a difference; then there was the whole 'peace and love' movement. He saw America as a place that believed that what young people had to say was important and that young people were entitled to their viewpoint.

'The biggest issue for American youngsters was the war in Viet Nam. For me it was a big issue as well because I thought: Here is a big powerful country, the biggest democracy in the world, bombing the shit out of some poor backward Vietnamese people. And sending young American boys off to die in stinking jungles in South East Asia. It was an intensely personal relationship, I think, for everybody who watched the war on television. We saw it nearly every night.'

There were rows again at home as John became-increasingly rebellious. He refused to get his hair cut and clearly enjoyed standing up to his father who by this time was working as a taxi driver in Dublin, and still gambling.

It was 1971 and the sixties were still big. It was a Brave New World and John felt part of this new feeling, this new sensitivity. He enjoyed getting stoned in Santry. There were lots of girls around, lots of cuddling and heavy petting, and occasionally full intercourse. His first experience of this was at thirteen with a sixteen-year-old girl from Santry. 'It was the usual fumbling but it was enjoyable.' Heavy petting was more usual because sex was always curtailed by the fear of pregnancy. There was an atmosphere of it being okay to express your feelings sexually. He remembers men hugging each other and feeling easy about it. That would have been taboo in working class Finglas. It was all fairly harmless compared to what was to follow.

During that year he read *Junkie* by William Burroughs and everything changed after that. The book is about heroin addiction and the descriptions of opiate hits in the book attracted John.

'So for the next couple of months I hung around with all my hippie friends, dropping acid, smoking hash and getting laid. But after reading *Junkie* I decided on a plan of action. I decided I was going to try opiates. It was quite deliberate. I was in the drug-taking milieu already but I'd never seen heroin, never seen morphine, never seen opium. I had never even seen anybody who took them. Most of the people I was with who used cannabis or acid or magic mushrooms, they were totally anti "smack". But not me. I was fascinated. I thought - this is something for me.'

At this stage John was into a network where drugs were swapped. He had access to grass which his mates grew and they swapped it for acid. One day while doing a swap he noticed that the guy he was swapping with was really stoned and he knew this was something other than acid. He asked what he was taking, thinking it was a tranquiliser. It was heroin.

'I said: "Wow, really. You don't know where I could get any of that." I was only just going on fourteen and this guy was about eighteen and he said I was too young. "What do you mean I'm too young?" I said. "I've been taking drugs since I was twelve. I'm not too young." But he said to let it go for a while.'

John let it go for a while until his fourteenth birthday when he had some money.

'I went up to this guy's house just where Finglas East becomes Ballymun and knocked on the door. He asked me in and we went upstairs. I'll always remember it. His brother was lying on a bed and his friend was lying face down on the other bed nodding out. And I just thought, Wow, this is for me.

'I said I wanted to buy some smack but they didn't have any. But they did have morphine, ampoules of morphine, and I thought, that'll do. He said I'd have to "fix" it, and I had never had a fix. I don't think I had even had an injection.

'I remember that Pink Floyd poster of pyramids that used to be in everybody's bedroom on the wall. On a little table there were three syringes laid out and beside them these little glass bottles which at the time I didn't know were ampoules. They had robbed a chemist and I thought, Wow, these are really cool people. I mean they're out robbing chemists. I've really lucked out here. These are the real people. I think what impressed me was they seemed so nonchalant. They seemed so sure of themselves. It was like: We have it sussed and everybody else is an asshole. And it went along with the feelings of uniqueness and strangeness that I had inside me, that I was destined for different things.

'I remember the guy saying that since it was my first time they had better just give me half an "amp" because "We don't want to kill you". I remember laughing and saying give me it all. He said: "No. You're only fourteen and I don't want you dying here in my bedroom."

'I've often thought about it, just how sick junkies are. You know, a fourteen-year-old kid comes in and asks for morphine or heroin and they say Yes. They had robbed a chemist so it hadn't cost them anything. They gave it to me for a present because it was my birthday.'

His fourteenth birthday was the first time John injected an opiate into his bloodstream. No one pushed

21

him to do it. He sought it out and if refused there he would have tried elsewhere until he got it. He was to continue injecting opiates for the next fourteen years.

Chapter 4

MORPHINE AND HEROIN

It is often said that addicts spend their lives trying to recreate their first hit. John remembers it all clearly He watched as the top was broken off the bottle. He remembers a little morphine being squirted out to clear out air bubbles and thinking this was a waste. He didn't know what a tourniquet was. He was shown how to fix a tie around his arm and flex his wrist to bring up his vein.

I remember from what I had read in William Burroughs that the prick of the needle is pleasurable itself. And it was. It felt good. It felt right. I remember he drew back the blood and I was fascinated looking at my blood running into the clear liquid in the syringe and mixing up in a kind of patterny swirl. And then he said he was going to start putting it in. I get an itch just thinking about it because you get itchy when you do morphine. I can feel it in the back of my neck even now.

He put it in and it was just incredible. First of all my whole body went warm. There was singing, that's the only way I can describe it, singing in my veins, flowing around from head to toe. And then suddenly this rush started in the small of my spine and shot up my spine and blew my brain out through the top of my head. I remember trying to get awake, trying to look around, and they were laughing at me because I was so stoned. I was all over the place. I was trying to speak and all I could say was: " That was lovely. Do it again!".

'I stayed there all day and had a second hit. It was the same as the first one except I knew what was coming and the anticipation made it even more pleasurable. The feeling that when the pain of the prick is over you are going to have the pleasure of the hit. You built up this anticipatory pleasure, almost sexual.

'When you take your first hit of morphine or heroin all your problems disappear. They vanish. You feel totally self-sufficient, self-aware. It makes you feel big, and capable. You feel like you have it sussed and wonder why isn't everybody doing this?'

The three seventeen- and eighteen-year-olds began discussing what to do with John. Should they let him call back or not? They did it for his birthday but said otherwise he was a bit young. He pleaded with them and eventually they agreed that he could come back but told him to keep it to himself. Of the four people in that room two are now dead and John has AIDS.

So John's first encounter with junkies was in a bedroom in Finglas East. He remembers the smell of stale unwashed bodies, incense and hash. And from that day on his life took two very different but parallel lines. He still kept up contact with his hippie friends, smoked grass and took acid. He was a 'peace and love' character who dealt in grass in a small way. But he also became involved secretly in hard drugs, skiving off unbeknown to his friends to a junkie pad in Ballymun.

He was still at school and to this day doesn't know how he kept going. For the time being his hard drugs were restricted to weekends. He did his Intermediate Certificate examination and got good results - three B grades five Cs and a D. They included a B in history. He had taken a tab of acid that morning and was tripping through the exam.

Most of the opiates available at that time were from chemist shops that had been broken into, so as a fourteen-year-old he had tried several types of morphine - Cyclomorph, morphine sulphates, Omnipom, Pethidine - all the ampoule-type drugs. He returned to the same flat in Finglas East, slowly increasing his visits to maybe twice a week as well as weekends.

'At the time it was easy to get prescriptions for dangerous drugs. Doctors were very lax then. The older guys would forge letters from hospitals saying that they had some incurable disease, usually cancer. This would be shown to a doctor who wouldn't bother to ring up the doctor whose name was on the letter to find out whether it was real or not. A very good one as well was supposedly having a sick mother. You'd go down with a letter from your mother and get a prescription. People could con most drugs from some doctors. Sometimes the prescriptions would be robbed. If they robbed a doctor's bag they would get prescription pads so they would forge a prescription and take it to some chemist down the country somewhere. They never checked to see if it was stolen. Once the prescription was cashed they would know that that chemist had a DDA - deadly dangerous articles box. Some people would break into chemists down the country and prise these boxes off the walls.

'I used go down to Finglas East and get morphine or Omnipom but they would keep the cocaine or smack for themselves. Then one day I went up and they had just robbed another chemist and they were just back from the country and they had loads of stuff and it was all over the bedroom. And I remember saying, "Can I have some smack?" and they said "Yes."

Pure pharmaceutical heroin, white diamorphine, was John's first contact with heroin. This is the heroin that is made legally by pharmaceutical companies and it is used for pain control in hospitals, usually for people with terminal illnesses. It was another major step in a relationship with drugs that was coming to dominate his life.

'One of the guys picked it up on a matchstick, a little matchstickful because it is so strong. You just put it into water and it disappears because it is chemically pure. By this stage I was just about able to give myself a fix, but I used to usually ask them to do it because they were so much better at it. But sometimes they would be so stoned that I would have to try and get it myself. I was chubby and fat and I could never see my veins. I used to have to feel them and then try and hold them and stick the needle in in the same movement.

'He gave me the smack, he gave me the works and said could I do myself. I said no, would he mind doing it, and he didn't mind because there is a sort of etiquette among junkies that you'll do somebody else's turn-on for them.

'Now morphine is a very zappy rush, very hot, very tingly, very intense. This smack was so smooth. It was like velvet, an iron fist in a velvet glove. He put it in and I remember saying: "Hey, this isn't like morphine. I don't feel... any... thing", and that was it. I remember my head going down between my knees and I remember just sitting there and waves of pure pleasure sweeping over me. They just come from your feet up and go through your whole body. I suppose starting with it spoiled me.

It is so smooth. It is like the Rolls Royce of heroin. Some people don't like it. They like a more morphine rush off their heroin, but I like my morphine to be morphine and my heroin to be heroin.'

Friends for life. John was captivated immediately by smack. To his way of thinking nothing else compared. Soon he was using every second day. It was simple straightforward swapping. He had grass which his friends grew. The Ballymun group robbed chemist shops.

Then about six months later he discovered Diconal which he still thinks of as his all-time favourite drug.

'I had often noticed that sometimes they'd have pink turn-ons but I could never figure out what it was. It was Diconal. Dic usually comes as a pink tablet and it is an extremely strong synthetic painkiller. I used to crush the tablet into a pink powder, use a lot of water because there is a lot of chalk in it, and inject. The rush off Diconal is not like anything else in the world. It is the strongest, zappiest, most "out of it" rush. It is like a mixture of morphine, cocaine and acid all gelling into a unique hit. And I loved it from the start. I absolutely adored Diconal. I think I must have done my first Dic when I was fifteen.'

John's lifestyle was quite routine.

'Go to school. Come home from school. Collect some grass. Sell some grass. Pay the guy who owned the grass. Get more grass and go down to my dealer friends. Swap some grass for smack, or whatever was available - Opium, Pethidine, injectible Valium, Diconal, cocaine, Palfium.'

This was 1973. They were a self-contained little scene.

The parents of the Ballymun brothers seemed to know what was going on but didn't do anything about it. Anything that went on in the bedroom was okay. And John had his parents trained as well. People scored grass from him in the bedroom of his house. His mother just thought he was very popular! Sometimes she used to bring up tea for ten people to the incense-filled bedroom. John still isn't sure how much she guessed. He thinks she was aware he was taking soft drugs but had no idea how far things had gone.

Of the Finglas East group John remembers them as very nice guys. 'They were really fucked up but I didn't know that at the time. One overdosed when I was seventeen. One was killed in a motorbike crash. And the other is clean now. They were the first casualties of drugs that I ever came across.'

Chapter 5

NIALL

The day after John's sixteenth birthday his brother Niall was born. Niall had spina bifida and wasn't expected to live. Now thirteen, he is confined to a wheelchair. When he was born the family was still living in Finglas. It was a tremendously difficult year for them, in particular for his mother.

'We were over the moon when I was pregnant. It was completely out of the blue. All of the gambling had passed. I took Jack to Gambler's Anonymous. I heard stories there. I thought I was bad!

'Then Niall was born and it was an awful blow. We didn't think he would live. Then I came home and the first year of Niall's life was spent sitting in the hospital. We were waiting for him to die and afraid to leave the hospital in case he did. That year I neglected the others at home. But there was no other way.

'And in that year my husband went back gambling. Oh God, he went back! And we decided to break up and did for a month. I just couldn't handle it. We went to marriage guidance.

'And in that year I cried a lot. People sat with me and cried. Now by this time John was nearly seventeen - and all that hassle. Maybe nobody gave him any attention.'

John's sister Avril remembers it well. She was eight at

the time.

'I can remember my Da coming home from the hospital and telling us we had a brother. Me and my brother Pat - we were on the stairs and John was in the hall. He was after sending us up the stairs for something. We were thrilled and wanted to know when it was coming home and my Da said: "Probably not. We'd have to wait and see." I remember that night John upstairs and he was crying his eyes out. He was like a baby.

'Two weeks later my Ma came out of the hospital. The following week the old fellow went missing. There was no money. The year after Niall was born was dreadful for gambling. He tormented us … gambling, gambling, gambling. My Ma used not even have her bus fare to go to the hospital. Only for our neighbours she would never have got in to see him.

'That year I didn't even get a coat for Christmas. I can remember it. Only John got us stuff that year we would have got nothing. He was working in a pub at night and he was doing a few bits in the markets. But my Da doesn't remember any of that. He has as bad a memory as John. They really have selective memories.'

All was not quite as it seemed to eight-year-old Avril. John was only occasionally working in pubs. The money was coming from other sources, mostly dealing in grass.

Chapter 6

THE MOST EXCLUSIVE CLUB IN THE WORLD

John's schizoid life between schoolboy, soft-drug hippie, and secret hard-drug user was by now becoming well established. After his Intermediate Certificate exam he moved into Form 5A, but the juggling act was becoming more difficult to maintain. A quick intelligence was no longer sufficient as the volume of schoolwork increased.

'Homework was becoming a major drag. I wasn't able to get through everything in school during the day. Also I wasn't going every day so it meant I had catching up to do. I still found it very easy except for a couple of subjects ... advanced Irish and advanced maths which I had a lot of problems with. But I had no time for doing homework so that anything that didn't get done during school hours just didn't get done. I was still able to prepare for exams by taking speed and staying awake all night. I could get essays in on time but the quality of my work was falling. The sheer volume that had to be done needed more commitment that I was willing to give it.'

And although he did not recognise it at the time his mind and personality were beginning to be dominated by drugs.

He remembers the contrasting environments he was

part of. The junkie pad was always filthy. There would be clothes strewn all over the place, a stale smell, syringes and broken ampoules lying around, and the bedclothes never seemed to be changed. By contrast the hippie bedrooms would be a bit untidy but scrupulously clean. The hippies had long hair, but it would be clean. His addict friends on the other hand had short tidy hair but were incredibly dirty. He remembers himself as being in between.

He would still join his hippie friends, talk hippie talk, still believe in getting out of Viet Nam, in 'peace and love' - tune in, drop out and take acid. Quite a few of his friends from school were also involved. There was a bit of hippie free love. Sex was never particularly important, but it was always there and easy. John had lots of hippie girlfriends and no one was much worried about commitment. Condoms weren't heard of. Nor was the pill. Pregnancy was still the big fear.

'Most of the hippie chicks were into pleasure themselves and into pleasuring people and it was great for someone like me. It was a kind of a fringe benefit. I remember when I was younger trying to get off with girls and it was so fucking difficult. There was this whole rigmarole involved where you had to go out and go to the pictures before you got a chaste little kiss on the cheek. I could never understand the Irish mating game. Acting out this bizarre ritual was beyond me. You had to play kiss-chasing for three weeks first. The hippie thing was more: "Hi, I'm John, what's your name? Do you want to have a joint?" And then get into some nice kissing and whatever else developed.'

Simultaneously there was this other need which only heavy drugs seemed to answer. Even at this stage drugs were beginning to diminish John's sex drive, but he didn't notice that until later when he took a break from opiates.

And it was taking its toll on his academic performance. They had been noticing in school.

'One teacher pulled me aside and said, "I don't know what you're doing but you'd better stop it because you're going to mess up your life." He tried to get it through to me that I had a bright future. It never crossed anyone's mind that it was drugs. They thought it was alcohol or home problems. Then just before the Leaving Certificate I got caught smoking grass at lunchtime and I was expelled. They let me back to do the exams.'

Just two years after a good Intermediate which got him into 5A he failed the Leaving Certificate miserably. His grades were one C, one D and one E, and he hadn't turned up for most of the other exams.

When he was about sixteen John began selling hash as well as grass. It was 1974 and it was the first time he had seen any more hash than would make few joints. Then it was a half-kilo slab and he was given 200gm to sell. He was at the end of a distribution chain and didn't even know who was bringing it into the country. By the time he was sixteen-and-a-half he was selling half a kilo of hash a week, which amounted to a lot of money. It was 75p a gramme at the time. He dealt fairly openly from a pub in central Dublin with diddle-e-eye music in the background. His clients knew where to find him after school. He couldn't rely on his parents for money. This way he had more than enough.

It was a busy but carefree time. Because there was

usually a gap of a day or so between shooting up, he hadn't yet got a physical habit. But he acknowledges now that he had developed a severe mental dependence. What does he think was happening?

'When you have a physical habit you need to shoot up every day, usually more than once a day, or else you become physically ill. You begin to physically withdraw. You lose control of your bowels, you sweat uncontrollably, you get pains in your joints. It is like an extremely severe bout of flu. And on top of that you know that the tiniest bit of heroin will make you better. There is a terrible psychological yearning and craving for the ease and peace that a fix will give you.

'At that stage I would have liked to take heroin every day. But if I didn't have it on a particular day I could still function. I would be thinking about it but I wouldn't physically need it to get out of bed.

'Some people say you're born to be an addict. Others say it happens to very sensitive people. In many ways I took the early stuff to kill the pain I felt. I felt the pain of uniqueness, the pain of being different, the pain of my father and mother constantly fighting, and by taking drugs I escaped from all that. Maybe only briefly, but I escaped.

'Part of me wanted to feel the same as everybody else but another part of me said, No, cherish this difference … you are meant to be different. And my active searching for an opiate drug after I had tried so many other drugs was a logical conclusion for me. I had to be different from even the people I wanted to be with.'

Nobody talked about addiction. Dublin didn't even have a real drug squad at the time. There were very few addicts and most of them were on the North side of the city in large Corporation estates. There were as yet no drug treatment centres. The drug legislation was just being tightened up. The main crime going on around drug abuse was the robbing of chemists and hospitals. It was petty crime compared to that of the late seventies and early eighties.

'Dublin was a cosy little place where all us hippies knew each other and all addicts just stayed quiet. I only knew of the three guys in Finglas East, about a dozen in Ballymun, and half a dozen in Finglas. Among ourselves we were proud of what we were. We were the people really living on the edge. We were "The Nazz". You know the David Bowie song from Ziggy Stardust: "We were the Nazz, with God given ass, came on so loaded man, well hung and a snow white tan." And I had still never seen anyone sick from junk because there was always enough around. There was always something to fix.

' There is a terrible sense of collusion between addicts, like: We've got the secret of the Holy Grail and you don't. And we would sit around talking about it and discussing the Grail. The Grail is drugs, and we follow the Grail and we give up everything for the Grail. The Grail gives us nothing back but we don't see that at the start. It gives us everything at the start. It heightens our feelings of difference. We're able to smirk at people and think, I know something you don't know. It's the most exclusive club in the world. We're a club and the cost of entry is your life. It is the most expensive club to join. You don't realise when you join but it is going to cost you everything you hold dear - family, friends and self respect.

'There is another song by David Bowie called "We are the Dead" and there is a line in that that goes: "Because of all we've seen, because of all we've said, we are the dead," and that is always how I have thought about addicts.'

Chapter 7

AMSTERDAM

John finished school with no plans whatsoever. Any thought about a job or career paled into insignificance beside his current life. He had more than enough money. He intended to continue more or less as he had been living, without having to spend daytime hours in school.

When a few of his hippie friends were going to Holland the summer after the Leaving Certificate he decided to go too. In the mind of every counter-culture person at the time, Amsterdam was paradise with its relaxed soft-drug laws, and the spirit of the movement with things like free white bicycles which everyone used. These were his soft-drug friends and he decided to stop fixing. Was this because he had become worried about his heroin use?

'No, I just decided that I was going to go to Holland and I was going to live differently. I was going to smoke lots of hash, take lots of acid, but I wasn't going to do any "gear". And it had something to do with the people I was travelling with, none of whom were into fixing.'

Holland was heaven for them. You could walk into a shop and buy hash. People smoked hash openly on the streets. It was legal to have up to about an ounce of hash for personal use. That is a few weeks' supply for a social user. There was a feeling of openness in Amsterdam in

1975 and it was everything most of them had dreamed of in a city. One of his school friends turned out to be gay and decided to 'come out' in Amsterdam where there was approval and plenty of opportunity. John wondered how to deal with it. It had never happened before and he wondered should he treat him any differently. But he soon came to the realisation that he didn't care one way or the other.

They lived in a big old farmhouse. The group was made up of a few of the well-to-do hippie friends from Santry that he had now known for about four years, a long-standing friend from Finglas, and some schoolfriends. And for the first time John got a 'proper' job. They all went to work in a flower bulb factory.

'It was hell. It was really hell getting up in the morning and going to work in a fucking flower factory. So pretty soon I started to retreat back to my old ways. I said I'd start getting the drugs for everybody. So we began getting into coke, speed, acid and hash in a big, big way. I had done a lot of speed but nothing like the way I did in Holland. And we were having to pay for it so I began working for this Dutch dealer - typical John! Find out where "the suss" is. Get in with the suss, and then start working for the suss.

'So suddenly I'm delivering hash all over Amsterdam … living with my friends outside Amsterdam, coming in every day and going to the Paradiso and the Milky Way and getting mindless stoned and lying there watching erotic movies. They had this cinema where instead of having seats they had beds. I remember going to my first porno cinema and having an old guy jerking off beside me.'

The sexual openness of Amsterdam in 1975 was amazing for any Irish seventeen-year-old. There was heterosexual permissiveness and homosexual openness and John remembers the blasé acceptance he felt when he walked into a dealer's flat to find him having sex with a young Malaysian boy. Anything was okay. In the mood of exploration John had a brief flirtation with another man, but rapidly decided that this wasn't for him.

John's drug use was out-of-hand within a matter of weeks. He didn't do much smack over there but he did do some. There was a lot of speed. So much that his four back teeth all fell out when he was eighteen from snorting speed. He was snorting pure sulphate which damages your gums and teeth and they just fall out. But the lifestyle suited him.

'Living there was wonderful. I'd get up in the morning and blow a chillum [a pipe of hash], have a wash, get dressed, go into Amsterdam, go and see the guys that I dealt for. They'd tell me what deliveries to make and I'd pick up the half-kilos of hash and strap them onto my body and deliver them all over the city.'

After a few months most of the original group that had travelled together went back to Dublin. John stayed on and went to live with three nurses. One was pregnant, a second had only one leg, and he dived into group sex with both of them with relish.

'Dutch women, there were no games. There was none of this three weeks of bullshit. It was: I like you. Do you like me? And I said Yes and the next thing I knew we were fucking our brains out like rabbits in bed. It was the first time I ever was involved in a threesome.

'Holland was great, living with these three women and going to the bars and I wasn't doing much smack. But of course I met a girl who was into smack and she was into me and whenever I was with her she would give me some. This was the first time that I had ever come across non-chemical smack. It was real organic heroin. All the stuff I had used in Dublin had been stolen from chemists.

'This was the first time I had seen brown heroin and the first time I "chased the dragon" - smoking smack. I couldn't do it and I was coughing it out, but, man, I got the hang of it pretty quick!

'Basically you have a number of major families of heroin. Heroin is refined from a morphine base which is made from opium. There are many different ways of cooking the morphine base into heroin. There is Pakistani, which is usually brown and it is one of the better smoking heroins, but it can also be injected. Then there is Persian, which is generally a slatey grey colour, or fawn. That is much better for injecting. There is Chinese rocks, which is pink heroin and is basically a smoking heroin. Then there is Thai, which is the nearest to pharmaceutical heroin that you get. It is usually white and very potent. The couple of times I have almost died have always been from white heroin. It is so much stronger than what you are used to.

'You get different feeling from each of them. I always liked either Thai or Paki. Some people like the Iranian. I suppose it is like drinking Scotch. People have their own preferences.'

Holland was a good time for John. He had good Dutch and Irish friends. He had a good time sexually. It was what he had left Ireland for and it lived up to all the expectations. But there was a gnawing feeling that something was missing, and that was drawing him back to Dublin. The feeling of strangeness, of not quite belonging, was rising up again.

And his drug distribution had got out-of-hand. He now occasionally set up heroin deals on his daily run. This brought him into contact with the tough end of the drug culture, something he had not encountered before. One day there was a misunderstanding over a deal and he found himself facing an angry Chinese man coming for him with a knife.

'It wasn't my fault. It was just that the punters had gone away. I had set up the deal and the guy had come along and bought half of what he wanted and said he'd come back for the other half but didn't. So your man was standing on the street corner when I came strolling along and he went for me. We used to fight a lot in Finglas but this was the first time anyone had actually tried to kill me. This guy really wanted to cut me up. He wanted to carve me into ribbons and it was a profound experience!'

Chapter 8

DEALING IN DUBLIN

After six months in Amsterdam, John was back in Dublin and rapidly into life as it had been before. He was dealing in hash again. But there was one important change. This was 1976 and it was the first time he had seen organic heroin in Dublin, and for the first time he had to pay for it. 'It was Chinese rocks.'

He also got a job in a clothing warehouse in Dame Street. This was simply to satisfy his mother, and most of the time he was so 'out of it' he fell asleep on the bales of cloth. He used to deal on Thursdays and Fridays and make about £300 from a kilo or a kilo and a half of hash, while bringing home £27 a week wages from the warehouse. He used to give his mother £50 a week, but she never asked where it came from.

He was an eighteen-year-old with loads of money who bought smack for himself. He kept his two separate circles of friends and didn't supply heroin to anyone else. The hard-drug scene was still small, but bigger than before. There was a drug squad and drugs were beginning to be noticed as a potential problem.

'A lot of people were using heroin and cocaine. There was a lot of Mescaline around. There weren't a lot of junkies but a lot of people were experimenting with heavier drugs. Where before I knew of twenty or thirty, now it was one or two hundred who were injecting or snorting whatever came their way. A lot of them never became junkies. It was all sorts of people. A lot of older hippies, younger hippies of seventeen and eighteen who needed something harder. It was the first time that I met really wealthy people, a lot of Southsiders who were heavily into coke and smack. People with very well off parents, lots of students, some UCD but a hell of a lot of Trinity.'

After about four months of keeping up the pretence of a job, he quit and moved in with a friend of his to a house which they called The Bunker. From now he was a full-time dealer in acid and hash from that house.

'Then I began to get a habit. It started slowly. I used to buy a day at a time. Then I began to buy enough for the weekend. And then eventually I began to always have some. Then getting to the stage of having it delivered. Then I remember waking up one morning and there was no smack and after about three hours I was in bits. I was puking, falling down, sweating, pissing myself, shitting myself. I hadn't realised that I had been building up a big huge habit. I was fixing about two or three times a day. I had never seen anyone sick. Not at that stage.'

Around the same time more Diconal came on the scene and John took the pills by the handful. And he had his first overdose on medicinal heroin.

'Some guys robbed a hospital in Northern Ireland and they came down to sell the gear to us. We used to make our initials in heroin on a mirror and snort it . I snorted J and half the M and overdosed. I remember waking up on people's shoulders being dragged around and my feet were dragging along the ground. They were whacking me keeping me awake. I nearly died. I was given mouth-to-mouth resuscitation. They didn't call an ambulance because it would have involved the police and this was a dealing pad.'

Things continued much as they were. He bought a motorbike. They had loads of money from dealing in hash where the profit was about £200 on every ounce sold. He never really thought about how much they were spending on drugs. There was always plenty of money in the house, so a hundred to the smack dealer wasn't noticed.

By that time there were four or five smack dealers in Dublin that John knew of. There were people robbing chemists, people conning prescriptions from doctors, and people forging prescriptions, or 'scripts' as they were universally known.

'We were dealing the hash for some very heavy people, two different gangs. One day one of the gangs came down and plonked an ounce of heroin on the table and said, "Sell that." They didn't say, Do you want it? They said "Sell it," and told us how much it was. They didn't know we were into smack, so we just used it all and paid for it out of our hash money. We did that for quite a while. But you can't keep that up for very long when your habit just keeps going up and up and up. Within about a year of coming back to Dublin I had a gramme-a-day habit and that cost eighty or ninety quid. That's fixing three or four times a day. I was a mega fuck-up. I was the sort of junkie that other junkies used to say, If I ever got as bad as you I'd stop.

'We were dealing away there and when the smack came it changed everything. We still had our hash people coming up, but we also had another crowd, and most of them were not hippies. They were town people from the inner city and from Finglas and Cabra and Ballyfermot, Killester, Neilstown, Coolock, Dun Laoghaire, Dalkey, Bray, Killiney, and students from Trinity and UCD.'

The average day began around 3 p.m. A fix started the day, then a joint and then some breakfast. Women were a non-event for John. He was purely into smack. People would arrive for hash. The house had double doors which opened out, and no one got in unless they wanted to let them in. They had a couple of hangers-on. One guy swept the floor and made the tea for a fix. Another opened the door for hash. It was like a little cottage industry. People usually came around tea time. Then came a major change.

'We started selling smack. It is as simple as that. We needed to to keep our own habits going. The only way to do that was by selling.

'What happened was that the organised gangs started bringing in smack before there was a market for it. So they created a market. They laid smack on people. They didn't take smack themselves. They were in it purely and simply for the money. They had made a lot of money out of hash and they saw an opportunity to corner a market that could only grow. I remember when that ounce of smack was thrown on the table thinking things are never going to be the same again.

'It was implicit that we either sell these drugs or get out of the country. These people were extremely heavy and had hurt people previous to this for much less than refusing to make them money. We were only about nineteen and didn't feel we had any choice. These were men in their mid-thirties with very violent reputations that we were dealing with. If they asked you to do something you did it. And there was protection in that when you were associated with these people other people were afraid to rip you off. You were looked after.

'For a while it was difficult to find people to sell the smack to. So we did it all ourselves. But after a while customers started to arrive. Mostly at the start it was the more adventurous of the ex-hippie types, including a couple of the Santry people.'

John graduated to two grammes a day, six or seven 'turn-ons'. He had also developed a taste for Diconal, which is an hallucinogenic as well as an opiate. Diconal also contains chalk and gelatin, which clog up your veins. He used to crunch up the tablets into a fine powder and dissolve it in water. If you miss the vein you frequently get an abscess. His arms were in a bad condition. He injected into his hands and fingers. He was into cocaine, and speedballs or highballs, which are coke and smack fixed together.

Then a wholesale chemist was robbed and the market was flooded with Diconal and Palfium. People who a week before were hustling small amounts of hash suddenly had opiates in their pockets.

'It was just crazy. I didn't realise what was going on. All I saw was that suddenly it was easier for me to get smack. I was in the throes of addiction and all I knew was that I needed a continuous supply of heroin. I never felt good about selling smack. Selling smack was a necessary evil. My intelligence had been put on the back burner. It was somewhere in the corner crying '.

Chapter 9

BUSTED

1978 was the first time John fell foul of the law. He had got away with it from the time he was twelve to when he was twenty. At the time he was living in a rented house in Lucan, outside Dublin, which happened to be owned by a policeman. A large number of police raided the house. Half-way through the raid the Garda who owned the house arrived and was comforted by his colleagues as they tore the house apart! The occupants were caught with a weighing scales, a few small pieces of hash, a small amount of heroin and a small bit of cocaine. Nine people were brought to Lucan police station and there were so many that they couldn't all fit in the cells, so they spilled over into the hall. It had elements of farce, but John was scared.

'I didn't know what was going to happen. It meant as well that my name was going into the newspapers and the parents would find out exactly what I was doing. It was a very traumatic time for all of us.

'All they wanted to know was who was supplying us and of course we wouldn't say. They were a bit angry but at that time the police were very nice. The smack explosion was only beginning to gain momentum.

'It was the first time I was ever in a police cell and I was charged with possession of hash. They did us all for dealing as well, but they dropped the dealing charges later. Normally when you are busted for any controlled substances you are charged with possession of the drug and with intent to supply. But if it is less than a certain amount, which the police seem to decide themselves, then they generally drop the dealing charge and just proceed with the possession charge and that was what happened in the Lucan case.'

Later they were in court in front of a travelling District Court Judge. They were legally represented and all nine sets of parents were there. The dealer who supplied them was at the back of the court keeping an eye on the proceedings. They all pleaded guilty to possession. John was fined £80 for possession and £80 for allowing the premises to be used for drug taking. One person found with heroin was fined an extra £50.

'It was crazy. He should have got a suspended sentence or something but the judge just lumped all drugs together.

'The first thing we did was go over to the pub across the road and have dinner. And we were nipping out to the toilet to have a smoke because we all had brought smack with us in case we got locked up. I had it up my bum in a bit of silver paper.

'I remember my mother saying to me, "I hope this is the last time I'll have to be in court for you." I remember thinking it probably wouldn't be.'

Chapter 10

ON THE CONTINENT

A few months later John decided to get away from
Dublin for a while and went to Cannes for the film
festival. His habit had reached the stage that he brought
an ounce of heroin with him for personal use. It was
enough to last about two weeks. He carried it in a powder tin and got through customs in Nice without any
problems.

There he met a stunning thirty-six-year-old American
woman at the airport. He helped her with her bags, and
that began a passionate affair that took them all over the
South of France, Italy and Germany for a few months.
Kathy (not her real name) had a lot of money and she
paid for his habit. For an addict that was heaven. She
didn't use drugs at all but was infatuated with John.
They lived in hotels and through the summer had one of
the main sexual relationships of his life. The business
was still going on in Dublin so he had money sent over
whenever he wanted it.

And for variety he worked as a gigolo in Cannes with
fifty- and fifty-five-year-old women. 'My dealer, who
was gay, and his boyfriend were two very handsome
young guys. They dealt some coke and smack on the side
but their basic business was providing escorts for older
women who had come to Cannes specifically for sex.

What happened was I owed them some money and Kathy was in hospital and I was waiting for money to come from Ireland and they needed an extra person so they asked me to do it. I did it twice. The first lot were from Dallas.

'The women told us exactly what they wanted. That was where I first learned what a "golden shower" was - pissing on "old ones". This woman asked three of us to piss on her. So she lay on a bed on a rubber sheet that she had brought with her just for this purpose and the three of us pissed on her. She paid us $750 each for a day.

'The second time we had brought fixes of coke with us that we skinpopped in the toilet so that we would be able to perform. There were three women from Houston, wives of businessmen, and we did it singly. Then we did it doubly. One woman with three of us. We did whatever they wanted. I was looking really well then. Suntanned and thin. The wasted addict look!'

Kathy wanted John to go back to America with her and get married but they parted in London and he headed back to the old routine in Dublin.

Chapter 11

TWENTY-ONE

By the time of his twenty-first birthday John had a serious heroin problem, compounded by damage to his veins from Diconal and Palfium. But he had a thriving business and he had money. To celebrate his birthday he hired rooms in the Crofton Airport Hotel, invited his friends and family, and supplied everything, including crates of champagne. He was an addict. He was a dealer. He was living the high life. And his family were completely fooled. His mother remembers the party well.

'He wasn't living here and he came down and invited just us. No aunties or uncles which is what happens in our family. Anyhow Jack and I bought him a bracelet and we went out with his brothers and sister. I said, "Who's paying for all this?" But he just said: "No hassle. It's all paid for." It was the weirdest party I ever saw in my life. We left about half-eleven. None of them were on this planet. There was a band playing. John was supposed to be the manager of this band. I believed all this. I thought he was travelling around everywhere with this band. And when he came home he would give the kids a fiver and they'd be over the moon. I thought he was doing well. I was bragging about him. He was doing marvellous as far as I was concerned. When you think of it afterwards you're so bloody foolish.

'He used to buy warehouse stuff in the North and I thought he had a good head on his shoulders even if he hadn't a regular job. He used to always say to me that Elvis Presley's mother would have nothing on me by the time he was finished.

'How could you not notice? I knew about the pot and I never saw him with anything but a cigarette until he came back here. But even then I remember finding a lemon and vinegar in a box under his bed one day and asking him what he was doing with it. "I like it on sausages, Ma," he told me. It was only afterwards when I started reading that I realised they were for sterilising needles and so on. '

But other problems were developing. To get a 'works' (equipment to fix heroin), was getting more difficult. Often there was only one set among five people. There were so many people using that it was difficult to keep up the supply. Most syringes came from diabetics, some of whom were addicts. The source had been chemist robberies, but that was becoming rarer.

'The way it would go in my flat was this. I was a full-time junkie so I would have a works. Somebody would come in and they'd buy some smack and I'd let them use my works after me. I'd get my hit together. Put the gear on the spoon. Put the citric, or lemon, or vinegar in. Put the water in. Heat it. Put a piece of cotton or cigarette filter in and draw it up and bang it up into me. All the person using it after me would do was squirt a drop of water through the works once and immediately start making up their own hit. The blood would collect in a ring where the needle fits on to the barrel. To clean it you had to take it apart and suck it out so you'd be sucking in other people's blood.'

John continued life as a junkie dealer living in Dun Laoghaire, Santry, Rathmines, Rathgar, Leixlip - all over the place. By moving regularly he kept one step ahead of the police. By this time John was beginning to realise that he was totally screwed up. He couldn't go over two hours without a hit of smack. Then there was another big robbery and cheap Diconal was available again.

'Man, I went for it and I started banging up twenty or thirty Dic a day and going around in a total haze. I lived on rubbish. I didn't eat dinners. I just ate chocolate all day long so I was really fat. I was getting really, really screwed up.

'I didn't really care. You knew there were junkie chicks to have sex with if you wanted. You had the "gear" so you could score sex whenever you wanted. Women just accepted it. A lot of women addicts treat their bodies as a commodity. They are something to be traded and swapped. It was that explicit: "Are you going to come home. I've some Dic at home." No problem. Home. Have a turn on. Into bed. Quick sex. Fall asleep. Wake up in the morning. Turn on each. Bye bye.

'I was so fucked up I was just looking after myself. My habit was out of control. It had become a real struggle trying to make all that money every day. The hash dealing was falling apart because I wasn't together enough to do it. The more money I made the bigger the habit became and I was always behind. I always owed more than I had. I had to do whatever was necessary to get the money to keep on using. And there was a guy I used to deal hash for and he said I could only deal if I didn't use smack. He came into a flat one night and found me with a needle in my arm and he went down and he got a shotgun and put it in my mouth and said he was going to blow my brains out. It was just to scare me. Then he just gave me a few slaps around the head. So I lost that connection.

'Then in 1979 I attended Jervis Street Hospital for the first time for detoxification. I think I was there five or more times over the next few years. Their idea of a detox was to give you Methodone for fourteen days which didn't really help unless you were totally committed. And most of the time the only reason I did it was because I had no money or I was feeling very sick or I had a court case. I think a little bit of me wanted to stop and I would keep making these efforts but they never lasted.'

Chapter 12

FAMILY LIFE

John always returned to his family now and again to touch base. In 1978 when John was twenty they sold the Corporation house in Finglas and moved to Ringsend near the city centre and nearer to each of their families. His mother was delighted to be back to their roots.

'It was a great help for us to move here. When we lived in Finglas, Jack never even hung a strip of wallpaper. I did all that. And when we bought this house it was just a little shack. People said we were mad. And Jack said he would work on it and I told him he couldn't build Lego. Then he studied it and he built on Niall's room and the bathroom and recently a dormer room. It was good.'

What she didn't know was the truth about John's lifestyle. She still finds it hard to understand how she didn't suspect.

'I didn't know John was a full-fledged junkie until he was twenty-two. That's very hard to believe. I knew he smoked pot and I always warned him that it was going to lead to something heavier. "Oh no, Ma. Here's a book." I read it through - *Pot: For and Against*. And he said they were going to legalise it in America. And he was off with bands and I got cards from all over the place.

'Then a letter came in the post addressed to John, and John is his father's name as well, so I opened it. It was from Jervis Street Hospital. I got a bit panicky and I ran down to my husband's sister and she said we'd go in to the hospital.

'I rang first. It was a woman. So we went in and I asked her what she wanted to see John for. I told her I knew John smoked pot but that he never did anything other than that. She let me ramble on and after about a quarter of an hour she took out a file. "Now," she said, "I'll tell you about John."

'She told me that John had been in there for detoxification five times and that he was a heroin addict. It was unbelievable. I couldn't explain the feeling and then I took to crying. She was very kind. She was more than kind because she knew I didn't know. I was very upset. "Mrs Mordaunt," she said, "don't blame yourself. There are thousands of boys would love their mother to come in here, to be interested in what is going on and what is wrong."

'Then little things came back to me. He would always have long sleeves on. He always had marks on the back of his hand and I'd ask him what happened. "Oh, I scraped it off the wall when I was getting the motorbike out." But it is only later on that it all comes back to you.

'He came down to the house the next day and I tackled him. "No, Mam, no." He denied it straight away. "John," I said, "I have it in writing. I've been to Jervis Street." Then he broke down and told me. But he still didn't admit how long he was on it.

'Later, when he was really off the drugs, Avril and I asked him where all the hiding places were. This was before the virus. He had a leather jacket with a string going around the bottom of it. We couldn't find anything in it. There were seven syringes around the bottom. I remember finding Diconal in the radio.'

Avril found drugs and needles under the carpet in her room. 'One night my Ma flushed what John said was eight hundred quid's worth down the loo. The minute she found drugs they just went down the loo. He used to hide them among my clothes. And on top of my wardrobe. He used to hide stuff in the hedge at the end of the road. And on the little shelf at the top of phone boxes.'

Avril was fifteen when she first realised John was a junkie. 'I didn't realise until my Mum told us. She was after having an unmerciful row with John and she pulled his two sleeves up and said: "There. Look at his arms. That's where all the money is gone." Because we were asking him where his motorbike was gone. We were always used to John having things and he was telling us that he had sold it and was buying another one.

'I didn't know it was drugs. Sometimes I used to think he was gone backward. He'd be just sitting there saying he'd love a few jelly babies or an ice pop. Then he'd get up in the morning and he'd be normal John.

'It didn't really click until later when he was back living with us. His hands were in bits. He was after injecting into the front of them and they were all infected. He used to tell us he was in a row and he missed a fellow and hit the wall. Of course we believed him. We thought he was a great fighter or whatever.'

Looking back, Avril wonders how she didn't realise earlier. 'I suppose when you're that age you have more important things on your mind. I was working. I don't think I really had any interest at that time. When he had money we thought he was managing a band. He'd throw us a few bob and we thought he was great. He always had the leather gear and a motorbike.

'I never really discussed it with him until I was about eighteen. Then I became very close to him. I'd stick up for him to the last, but he caused more rows. They'd always be my fault, or my Ma's fault or my Da's - never his!'

Having John living in the house had a serious effect on Avril's teenage years. 'Apart from the rows, I couldn't bring my friends in. To get to my bedroom I had to go through John's bedroom. I don't know how many times I walked in and John would be lying there stark naked, maybe with an injection in his arm, or in the sole of his foot. I wouldn't take the chance. I caught him one day when he had no drugs just drawing his blood out into a syringe and pushing it back in again.

'Another night I was sitting on the couch with my friend and he came down the stairs wearing a leather jacket, white socks and a pair of underpants and that was it. He was hallucinating. My friend was on her knees laughing. She thought he was drunk. She didn't know.

'It got so bad that if I went out with my mates to a dance I'd ring and find out if he was in bed. If he was in bed I'd bring them in for a cup of tea. But I wouldn't bring a fella home. My social life was ruined because of John. I'd be going out with somebody and they'd be local and know where I lived and I'd say, "No, I'll meet you at the corner." I wouldn't let them call to the house.

'My feelings were never brought into consideration, ever. Especially where John was concerned. He used to say that I was all right. That was all he ever said. I had no problems. I used to say, "But John, you're my problem."

'The house was never our own. There might be two

58

fellows in the sitting-room and he'd be upstairs with someone else. I used to think he was pushing, but they were bringing it to him. Or so he says. He had millions of friends when he was a junkie.'

His mother remembers coming back one day and finding two friends of John's under Avril's bed. That night Avril found two syringes congealed with blood under her pillow. 'I freaked that night. I threw them at him. John didn't care once he was shooting up.

'Then my Da put his foot down and said that none of John's friends were to be allowed in. This was when we knew he was a junkie. We wouldn't take phone calls for him. We told everybody he didn't live here.

'John never got on with his father. I don't hit it off with him either. We kind of clash. But I do love him because I remember the good times with him as well as the rows about gambling.

'John does blame my Da for getting into drugs as much as he did. I mean I had to listen to worse rows than John ever had, but my Ma depended on me too much. And I do personally think that John might have a point in blaming my Da. Because John was never one that could cope with hassle. Even now he can't. He would tell you that himself. But my Da wouldn't accept that.'

John's mother thinks there is probably something in this theory too. 'We never had physical rows, but arguments. Maybe that had a lot to do with John. He said to me: "Ma, you used to think I was asleep. I'd be up in the bedroom listening to you." Especially the year Niall was born. Jack was gambling and I had all this worry about my child dying.

'I think John does blame his father a bit. Jack's attitude to John was - pull yourself together. As I said to him one night: "You above anybody should understand. You needed help too." John said to me once: "Ma, do you think I like being a junkie? Do you not think I'd love to get up in the morning and not know I have to."'

But irrespective of rows and hassle, his mother always preferred to have him at home. At least she knew where he was.

Chapter 13

COLD TURKEY

John's mother was willing to try anything at this stage.

'He came down here one morning and he was really ill and I made him stay. He was very depressed. "Mam," he said, "I feel rotten, and I feel rotten about what I'm after doing to you." I said it didn't make any difference and asked him would he do a "cold turkey" with me. I read everything about it and I had him in the parlour there. My own doctor came up and he was a brick. He came every night and gave him an injection. I don't know what it was but he was very understanding and he gave him great help. We helped him through from Monday to Saturday. He was weak, vomiting, up the walls. It was dreadful. We had to wash him. We sat with him twenty-four hours a day. But, and you'll find this hard to believe, on the Saturday night John wanted to go out and I knew if he went out he would inject. I asked him to give me phone numbers and I would go out and get him pot. I was willing to do that just to keep him from going out and injecting. Maybe he'd be found in a flat somewhere, dead.'

Avril, who was sixteen at this time, was helping. 'He wasn't too bad for the first two days. He was cranky and crabby. But then the third day it was terrible. He was screaming and roaring and convulsing. I was kind of frightened of him. It was a horrible experience. He would sweat and shiver. He'd go from a cold sweat to roaring the house down. He hated everybody and everything. He didn't want clothes near him or bedclothes. Then he'd be freezing and want them back.

'It was horrible. That's when I really knew what John was. I still loved him, but did you ever love somebody and not like them? I hated him, but I loved him because he was my brother. I told him. I said, "John, I love you but I can't stand the person you are."'

Then on the Sunday morning Avril noticed that he was all yellow. His mother rang the doctor. 'By that time he was frothing at the mouth. She was told to keep sugar in his mouth. The doctor arrived and diagnosed hepatitis. He took him off in his own car and had him admitted to Sir Patrick Dun's Hospital.'

John spent over three months in hospital and from now on hospitals were to be a regular feature of his life. The hospital knew he was a drug addict and maintained his addiction with Phiseptone.

He was seriously ill and his parents were sent for twice as the hospital thought his life was in danger. He improved after a few weeks, and, unbelievably, began dealing from the hospital. He was in a private room and people would throw the money up to the window and he threw the drugs out. He couldn't fix because they were checking his arms but he smoked hash in the toilet. Fairly soon he got caught passing drugs out the window, so he was moved to another ward.

As he was recovering from the hepatitis John developed an eating disorder. He lost weight rapidly and went down to eight stone, a large drop from his normal weight of eleven stone or more.

'There was something wrong in my head. I couldn't eat. I just couldn't do it. I got progressively weaker and weaker. My parents used to visit me nearly every day and they would bring my favourite food to try to get me to eat.

'I felt safe in the hospital. Phiseptone made sure I wasn't sick and I was getting in hash and some heroin, so I was quite content.

'The hospital were at their wits' end. They started feeding me on high calorie food and all the build-up stuff that old people eat. They used to show me the women anorexics to try and impress on me what I was allowing to happen to myself. But I felt I had no control over it. I didn't want to eat. I had no desire for food. In a way it was because I didn't want to get out of hospital, I think. I know I was really really pissed off with what I was doing but I couldn't see a way out of it.

'Then I started drinking and slowly they replaced the 7-Up with protein drinks and build-ups and it was a long slow battle. Getting back up to eight-and-a-half stone took ages. I think I had gone down to seven-and-a-half. It was only after I got over that threshold that I began eating again.'

Chapter 14

FEEDING A HABIT

After a long convalescence John returned to his parents' house at his mother's insistence.

'He was great for about six months. He was off drugs. I knew. I checked him. It was like a military barracks here. I checked his room. I checked his arms. Then he came in one day with his arm in a sling. He told me he fell and sprained his arm. It must have been my suspicious mind and I said, "Come here and I'll have a look at it." "Don't Ma," he said. "Well you bastard," I said. "You're injecting again, John." There was a big hole in his arm. And then he went on and on and on. Heroin wasn't enough. Nothing was enough until he eventually started taking Diconal. By Jesus when he took Diconal he was a madman.

'I had him living here and he'd go off. He'd be missing for two days. I always remember someone throwing themselves off a balcony in Ballymun and they hadn't been identified. I was fully convinced it was John. I was going to be real brave and go over. We rang and it wasn't him. But I was sure. Once he turned the key in the door at night I slept because I said if anything happens him or if he dies he's in a clean bed.'

Things went from bad to worse. Up to now he had always had money and had been reasonably healthy.

Now he was on the street with a monster habit and no dealing business to support him.

He spent six months shoplifting, a period which he describes as one of the worst of his life.

'I used to go out in the morning with a big shoulder bag, go down to Eason's, the Paperback Centre - all the bookshops. They got to know me after a while. I'd steal hundreds of pounds worth of books. I must have robbed hundreds of copies of *Life on Earth*. I used to sell them to all the different second-hand booksellers. It got so bad I was bringing them in three and four copies of the same book! They didn't bat an eyelid. They knew I was a junkie. They didn't care where the books came from as long as they had no stickers on them. I'd be in toilets peeling the prices off all these books.

'By this time the drug scene had hit the streets in Dublin in big way. You could buy "10-bags" of smack anywhere. A 10-bag is a little envelope, about half the size of a postage stamp, with heroin in it. It is just a piece of paper folded over and sold for £10. About twenty 10-bags made a gramme. You could get them in O'Connell Street, on Grafton Street, in practically every block of flats in the centre of the city. For me this was the pits because I had been used to using grammes of gear and then to have to spend my hard-earned fifty or sixty quid on six 10-bags was the pits. I hated it. Going out sick every morning, robbing, getting enough money to have a small fix, do more robbing. It was just fucking horrible.'

He nearly got caught in Veritas bookshop one day. They had just begun to employ security men in all of the bookstores. He escaped into a taxi, and lay on the back seat and told the driver he was trying to dodge a girlfriend.

Then just before Christmas he was caught shoplifting in Brown Thomas. He was marched in handcuffs down to Pearse Street police station. He remembers the humiliation well. He was in court on Christmas Eve. 'The judge asked if I had any previous convictions. I told him I was unemployed and I was shoplifting for Christmas presents. He fined me and gave me the Probation Act because it was Christmas. As soon as he let me out I went back and shoplifted again.

'Christmas for a junkie is the worst time of the year because Christmas day you usually cannot score. You can't even get out of your fucking house unless you've a car. I had a motorbike for getting out to doctors.

'One of the things that was to make my life really easy - and really hard too - was that I got some forged prescriptions for Diconal and I began passing them in chemists. Then I began going to every crooked doctor. We would get prescriptions for 100 Diconal and 100 Palfium. Now somebody with terminal cancer would be lucky to get 100 Diconal for a week or two. We were getting them every day.

'You'd find out where there was a "quack" and pay half your first script to whoever introduced you. Or sometimes twenty quid. I travelled all over the country to crooked doctors. Sometimes we would bring a woman. There were always doctors willing to write scripts for sex, for money or for whiskey. I remember going all over Dublin and all over the country. If you knew where to look you could always find an alcoholic doctor or a doctor who was into sex. I remember once nearly having to give a guy a hand job myself. He was touching me up and I thought: How far is this going to go? I really can't do this. Then he said, "You seem like a nice boy" and gave me the prescription. There were a couple of junkie doctors as well who had totally messed up their practices.'

Between 1981 and 1983 the drug scene in Dublin became serious criminal business. One gang operated in the Talbot Street area, selling 10-bags from ten in the morning. All the peace and love was well and truly gone. Now it was dog-eat-dog.

'People would knife you for a 10-bag, whereas before I used walk around with a quarter ounce, that's enough for 150 or 200 10-bags, in my pocket. If you did that in 1982 or 1983 you'd be likely to get your hand chopped off.'

The average age of junkies was getting younger. John remembers scoring off a ten-year-old kid who was stoned out of his head.

'He was the youngest brother of about six in a family that were all dealing. What happened was that the police got to know them so well that the older brothers couldn't do it. So the youngest brought the smack and nobody ever ripped him off because if you did the older ones would get you. Then he got into it himself. I think he's dead now. As is now well known whole families with mothers, fathers, brothers and sisters were involved.

'I remember one time getting a job. This guy I knew was supplying about fifteen little dealers with their bags of 10-bags and how it used to work was you'd get thirteen for the price of ten. Sell ten and three for yourself. What people did was they took the three and then hustled out to try and sell the other ten! I worked for a few weeks as a pack maker. Making up hundreds of packs was quite a laborious task. I'd sit at a table in a boarded up flat and chop it up. It'd take hours and you'd stop and fix every now and again. Now the beauty of this was you could skim some so you made the packs the same size but you cut it a tiny bit. You could cut it with lots of inert powders, usually with medicinal glucose that you could buy at a chemist. Or you could use natural unscented talc. People wouldn't buy it if it smelt. You had to get twenty-five 10-bags out of each gramme, and a gramme cost about £120, so the profits were huge. You skimmed off maybe a gramme out of each seven grammes. Nobody noticed. Everybody was into size, not quality. The whole city seemed to be dealing at various levels.'

By now some of John's friends from his early life in Finglas had got heavily into heroin. People were robbing anything they could get their hands on to swap for smack. There was a barter economy. A video was worth ten or fifteen 10-bags, cameras were popular, as were walkmans, radios, watches and especially jewellery.

John was doing a little dealing, generally hustling, and going to doctors for scripts.

'It was then that I began to get really bad. Banging up in toilets in town because you were so sick you couldn't wait to get home. Banging up in the street because you just had nowhere to go, in the stairwells of the flats. Paying 50p to go into somebody's pad, paying a pound to borrow a works for a quick fix. 'The quality of the heroin we were using was terrible. It was really cut to ribbons and around this time people started to die. What would happen was people would get used to buying 10-bags and then suddenly somebody would get in some good gear and put out some quarter grammes. Somebody would buy a quarter gramme and think it was only four 10-bags and it might be as good as ten 10-bags and they would overdose. I lost three or four people in 1983, and again in 1984.

'I remember meeting a friend of mine in a pub at nine o'clock one evening and he was drunk. He asked me to score and I knew enough about heroin and alcohol together to know he was too drunk to take any gear. So I refused to get it for him and so did a couple of other people. Of course he found somebody who needed a turn-on for themselves. I came back to the pub in Rathmines at a quarter to eleven and they were wheeling him out from the toilet. He went in, had a turn-on, and died. He was only twenty and I really liked him. He was gone. Dead.'

Chapter 15

CARLA

John had always been interested in motorbikes and had usually owned one which was useful for getting around the city quickly. Then he had the first of two crashes, neither of which was his fault, and each of which brought substantial monetary compensation.

'The first crash happened in the rain in Dorset Street. I was riding a Kawasaki 250 and a car from Monaghan took a wrong turn and hit me and smacked me into the path. I hit my chest and finished up in hospital. I woke up next morning and I was bringing up loads of blood. It turned out that I had damaged all the cartilage along my chest on the left hand side and I had a haematoma on my lung.'

No irreparable damage had been done. About the only good thing in John's life at that time was an Italian woman called Carla (not her real name). She was a junkie too but they had managed quite a long relationship in Dublin. They also lived in Italy for a while, two junkies together.

'We loved each other but it finished up badly. I nearly died in Italy from a thing called Toxic Shock Syndrome. Her parents broke us up. They were very wealthy and they offered to pay off all the debts I had built up in Italy to get me back home. Carla was supposed to come with me but her mother tried to commit suicide before we left, and we had a big tearful scene at the airport.

'She was a wonderful girl, but she was an addict just like me. It's a very tough relationship living with another addict when you're using. She would sit at home all day banging up gear while I was out hustling for us. It led to resentment.

'And to have proper sex we'd have to have coke because you couldn't function otherwise you'd be so stoned. It was a dead weird relationship, but I loved her and she loved me. We cared about each other immensely, but then, you're an addict. You're never sure about your feelings at all when they change so radically from day to day.'

John's mother remembers this time well. It was not long after she had learned he was using heroin. 'When that romance went wrong he started using very very heavily. She was a lovely girl but they weren't good for one another because she was in the same boat as he was. She was a junkie too.

'John would always tell me things. We have a great relationship. We're the kind of family - with all our problems, maybe some people would call us a problem family - but we all love one another. No matter what happened I always told them I loved them.

'When Carla lost their baby he told me. I felt so sorry for him when her parents took her back. But they were just trying to help her. She was a lovely kid. His life really went down then. He'd say to me: "But I love her, Ma. I'd even marry her." I'd say, "Don't do her any favours, John."'

Chapter 16

HOSPITALS

Carla had gone, acquaintances were dying because of drugs, but all this had no effect on John's using. He knew he was being watched by the police. He was having trouble with his parents and with many of his friends. He began to lose contact with some of his older friends. All he talked about was smack and they just weren't interested.

Gradually he began to deal again and it was good times once more as far as he was concerned. He still used large quantities of Diconal and needed three prescriptions a week from doctors. He became known as 'Pinkie John' because he always had Diconal. But it didn't last.

'I finished up in Baggot Street Hospital for an overdose. I finished up in St Stephen's for an emergency operation for another abscess. I finished up in Patrick Dun's for an emergency operation for an abscess. I finished up in Baggot Street for a clot in my leg. Hospitals were now a major factor in my life.

'It was a sick time. The city had gone sick. People were ripping people off, people were getting shot and getting knifed, babies getting kidnapped and held for ransom for smack. Some real scumbags started to drift into the scene. By 1984 the whole thing was fucked up.'

John was dealing enough to keep his habit going. But

he was plagued by deep venous thromboses (DVTs) as a result of injecting Diconal for such a long time.

'Usually the way it would happen was that my leg would begin to swell and go red. Then I would suffer the most incredible pain. I have never felt pain like I have felt from deep venous thrombosis. Sometimes I passed out. I was stabbed once in the shoulder and that instant of pain was what a DVT felt like all the time. It would take a week or more in hospital for the clot to break up.'

He had begun to use his groin to fix because his feet and arms were in such a mess. At one stage he had a needle strapped into his groin for ten days and carried a bottle of anticoagulant to break up the clots that formed in the syringe. He collapsed with septicaemia.

He was caught again by the police in Rathmines with a small amount of heroin and some hash. This was the first time he was charged with possession of heroin. He got off with a suspended sentence and a fine. Again he got a fright.

He continued to go to Jervis Street for two weeks at a time to detox. He thinks he went about thirteen times.

'They were worse than useless for me, but they allowed me to recuperate a bit because I wouldn't have to hustle for my gear for a while.

'I can't describe how squalid using had become. I remember using in a pad while a girl was shooting up underneath her breast while another guy was using his neck and I was sticking a needle in my groin. And it made no impression on me. This was just natural. Three people sticking needles into parts of their bodies that shouldn't ever have seen a needle.'

And he had a second motorbike crash about nine months after the first one. It happened near Crowe's pub in Ballsbridge. I was parked at the traffic light and it turned green and a guy broke the light coming across me and ran straight over me. The guy nearly got sent to prison over it. There was a criminal case as well as a civil case. My arm and leg and foot were broken and I was treated in St Vincent's.'

Accidents apart, by 1985 he was sinking. He was using about two hundred Diconal a week and was plagued by abscesses and DVTs. He used as much smack as he could afford. The police were searching him regularly. They weren't very interested in him personally. They wanted information on the people he had worked for.

'I wouldn't tell them what they wanted to know and they were saying that everyone else was ratting so why wouldn't I? It was mostly fear. If I had ratted on the people I had worked for I'd be pushing up daisies. I didn't work for the scumbags. I worked for the heavies.'

He was on crutches by now because his legs were in such bad condition from injecting Diconal. He was back living with his parents.

'My mother couldn't understand it. She just felt helpless because nothing she could do or say made any difference. She never threw me out because she knew that by having me there at least I'd get food and clean clothes. I was programmed for self destruct.'

He had been busted again with hash. Around this time the drug squad began using young undercover policemen to infiltrate the drug scene. They became known throughout Dublin as 'The Mockeys'. John was one of their early arrests in Christmas week 1984. It happened in a friend's house in Dorset Street. The police were dressed up as gas inspectors and had been watching the flat for days. John arrived to score some smack and one of them opened the door. John was caught and spread-eagled with a gun at his neck. 'They were a new breed of copper. They were the breed who watched Hill Street Blues. They never forgot about me after that and they made my life a torture.'

The police took a lenient attitude and told him he had better start to get his life in order. He decided to try the Coolmine Centre for drug rehabilitation. 'I was defeated and it was the only game in town.'

Coolmine faced an impossible task. Drug addiction is notoriously difficult to deal with. And addiction takes many forms. There are addicts who work and are clean during the week and fix at weekends. During the week they are okay but if they are without heroin at the weekend they are up the walls. Most addicts try many times before successfully quitting drugs, and those that do quit often say that you have to feel ready to stop. John was definitely not ready at that stage. He remembers Coolmine as a tough place which was based on the concept of tough love.

'Coolmine is a therapeutic drug-free community in Navan, County Meath. To get into it you have to be detoxified and when you arrive the first thing they do is search you and all your clothing completely. When I arrived they put me sitting on a bench where nobody was allowed to talk to me. There were people walking by that I knew from the streets but no one would speak to me. Then I was brought up before a panel of people made up of a member of staff and people further along in the programme. That initial interview was one of the heaviest things I have ever been through. They told me I was a thief and a liar and so on. Eventually I broke down and it was when I cried that they finally said they would admit me. It was to see if I had any commitment towards recovery. They say you have got to make an investment in the programme before the programme will make an investment in you.

'I was put in a dormitory with twelve people, with my own bed and locker, and that was my space to keep clean. I had to learn to make a bed properly. I had never done it before.

'There was a strict hierarchy depending on how long you had been there. I was put working in administration because I was quite sick and I could read and write well. You weren't allowed to do what was called "neggie rapping". You weren't allowed to talk about life on the streets. You weren't allowed to talk about drugs.'

John was a psychological disaster, he had to use crutches to get around and he stopped eating again. Anything he did eat he vomited up. After a few weeks at Coolmine he was getting progressively weaker. He was taken from there to Our Lady's Hospital in Navan and clinical anorexia was diagnosed.

'That was the first time I was fed on a nasal drip. I couldn't even hold down milk and water.' The hospital phoned his parents.

'We got a phone call from Navan Hospital to get down as soon as possible so Jack and I went down on a Sunday morning. John weighed six-and-a-half stone, from a fifteen-stone bloke. It was unbelievable. We were told to bring a spoon and a dish and some food and to try and get him to eat. We stayed with him as long as we could.

I brought him down things that I made, but no way. The sister said he would die.'

Gradually he began eating enough custard and jelly to maintain his weight and was released from hospital. While in the hospital he phoned a friend he had been 'doing scripts' with and got him to come down and together they found a doctor and got a script for Diconal. That was the end of rehabilitation for the time being.

While he was there a blood sample was taken and unknown to John he was tested for HIV infection.

He refused to go back to Coolmine and once back in Dublin he went on the streets for a few days before going back to his parents house in Ringsend where he would be looked after. Then he resumed active addiction with abandon using up to three hundred Diconal a week. His whole life again revolved around getting the money to get his 'scripts' and having the time to fix Diconal. There was nothing else in his life.

'I'd wake up in the morning. I would crush some Diconal in a piece of cardboard, dissolve it in a glass of water and inject it into my groin. That was before I got up. Then my friend would collect me and we would go and do some chemists and go to a house and bang up. I might do forty or fifty during the day and then come home at night.'

A few weeks later he finished up in St Vincent's Hospital with yet another deep venous thrombosis. The treatment for DVT is an anti-coagulant called Heperin. It is administered on a drip intravenously to break up the clot. Everything was fine. They went through his medical history and looked after him well, got him better and let him go.

Another few weeks and he was back in St Vincent's

again in the same condition as before, with yet another DVT and abscesses. He was put in a ward and was given the same treatment.

'Then after about a week or ten days they just came in one morning and they said they couldn't treat me any more. You have to go, now. I had bad diarrhoea at the time and I was still on Heperin. They told me I was going to Jervis Street and I would be looked after there. They gave me three letters and ordered a taxi. I thought this was really weird.

'So I arrive at Jervis Street, and they won't let me into the main hospital building. They send me around to the junkie prefab. I can't walk so I have to be carried in. I sit there in my pyjamas and my tracksuit bottom and a doctor comes along and he brings me into his office and tells me they are not taking me. I said that Vincent's had said that they would.

'I had met this doctor once or twice before. He had seen me and given me a detox once, I think. We had had a bad time together - he seemed to feel that I was just a fucked up junkie who had no chance of recovery. He didn't seem to think I had any interest in getting better.

'I rang my mother and told her what was going on so she came in with my aunt. I was running to the toilet every five minutes with this diarrhoea.'

Mrs Mordaunt remembers the incident well.

'The doctors in St Vincent's said that Jervis Street had agreed to take him and detox him. Now this was 1985 and we didn't know anything about the AIDS virus at the time. I said we'd take him to Jervis Street but they said it was no problem. So I was back sitting here at home and I got a phone call from Jervis Street to go and collect my son. I said he was an in-patient. They said they weren't taking him. "You have to take him," I said. But they told me he was sitting in the hall and to come and get him.

'I asked to be put through to a doctor and in the meantime my sister-in-law was here and she is one of those people who knows everybody and she said she would get in contact with our TD [Member of Parliament], so she contacted his secretary and he got on and so forth. So I got on to the doctor and said that if they didn't take my son out of the hall I was coming up and bringing the press with me.'

But that threat didn't have any impact. Mrs Mordaunt was shocked at this treatment, but the relationship between doctors and drug addicts is not an easy one. By their own admission most drug addicts are manipulative people - and good at it.

'I got back on to St Vincent's and said: "In the name of God what are you doing? You told me there was a bed." And they told me John had run away.

'They had put him into a taxi, wearing a tracksuit bottom and a pyjama top and with an incontinence sheet. When he got to Baggot Street Hospital he told the driver he would have to use the toilet. He was so sick he took a long time and the taxi driver came in looking for him and one of the nurses said he was in the toilet. The taxi then brought him to Jervis Street.

'I was too upset to go. I sent Avril in with a leather jacket and she took him home.'

Avril remembers going in on the bus and getting a taxi back. 'And as soon as he was in the door he plonks on the chair and starts giving orders. Like Hitler. Ring this person. Ring that person. That's when I had an inhuman row with him. I told him what I thought of him.'

Looking back, his mother's conclusion is that Jervis Street knew, St Vincent's knew and Navan knew that John was HIV positive, or 'body positive'. 'Everyone knew except us.'

The doctor did however agree to continue John's detox programme on an out-patient basis, which meant travelling to hospital every day, sick as he was.

Chapter 17

MORE HOSPITALS

Another few weeks passed and John was back to the same vast quantities of Diconal which he injected into his groin. Then he got yet another DVT and and abscess in his groin so he went back to St Vincent's.

'The casualty officer saw me and said they would admit me immediately. Next a consultant or registrar arrived and there was some dispute about whether I would be admitted or not. I couldn't figure out what was going on. A nurse came in and held my hand and told me not to be worried, that everything would work out. Eventually they came and said they couldn't admit me but had arranged for me to be admitted to Baggot Street Hospital. The nurse was crying. She gave me the taxi fare - I think it was her own money - and told me to go to Baggot Street.

'Baggot Street took me in. They put me straight in and put me on a bed. They didn't make me sit on a chair because a couple of the nurses knew me at that stage. But of course a few days after the abscess started to go down and the DVT began to disappear I was ringing up my Dic man again. He came up and collected me from the hospital and we went off and scored.'

John couldn't understand the behaviour at St Vincent's Hospital. He assumed it was because he was a junkie. The truth was much worse as he was soon to find out. He went back home again, where his mother was in despair. She remembers the end of 1985 as a dreadful time.

'He got worse and worse and my God he got so sick. It is unbelievable how sick he got. His friends brought his fixes when I was out. I know they did. The district nurse came and he wouldn't come out of his room. She went up to see him and recommended him to the Rutland Centre. We had an interview but they couldn't take him for another three months. He had to use a stick at the time. His legs and his groin were in bits. His toenails were coming off from injecting into his toes. I honestly don't know how he is alive.'

Meanwhile John was injecting huge amounts of Diconal and causing havoc in the house.

'You hallucinate on Diconal and one day I came down the stairs wearing just a leather jacket with a syringe sticking out of each groin talking to a friend that wasn't there. My mother just turned me around and brought me upstairs and pulled the syringes out of my legs and threw them away.'

She thought he had overdosed. 'I rang Jervis Street and they said to get Blanchardstown Hospital who were on call. I must have been really down in the dumps. I went up with a basin of water and disinfectant and cleaned him up. Then I took I don't know how many sleeping capsules and put them into a drink and gave them to him. I didn't intentionally want to kill him, don't get me wrong. But I couldn't take any more and I couldn't see him going any longer. I was thinking, Please God he'll be dead in the morning and he'll be at rest and we'll be at rest. My main thought all the time was if he was dead I would know where he is. When they are out you are thinking they're in an old flat now and they are injecting themselves. Every time I heard of somebody found dead in the toilet of a pub I'd say, "That's my John." Someone found dead in a flat, "That's my John."

'He slept until one o'clock the next day. I sat at the end of the stairs and I kept going in and looking at him and I said a few prayers. Then I took a tablet myself and went to sleep hoping it would be the end of a nightmare.'

Chapter 18

HIV POSITIVE

It was coming up to Christmas 1985 when John began to notice he was getting sick. He lost about three stone in as many weeks. He began to get very pale and breathless. Christmas passed off without event.

Then in January 1986 he had to see a doctor about injuries he had received in the motorbike accident in Ballsbridge.

'He was a consultant from Patrick Dun's Hospital. I arrived at his surgery. He just had one look at me and said, "You had better get up to the hospital NOW."'

John went straight home and told his parents. He got some clothes together and his parents took him to Sir Patrick Dun's Hospital which was just around the corner from where they lived.

'John couldn't walk and could barely breathe. He was put in a wheelchair to go the length of the corridor. They put him into a little side room. It was a Thursday. And they were very kind to him. I won't deny that.'

John doesn't remember much about the next day or so. 'They were giving me loads of Dic because I began withdrawing like crazy. They had to find out what I was on and give it to me to stop me withdrawing.

'After a day or so people began wearing gloves, masks and gowns and these full body-suits, and there was a nurse stationed outside my room at all times. They were giving me blood because they said I was anaemic. Then I developed shingles and thrush. I just thought, man I'm very sick. I was really out of it. I was so weak and so lack-lustre that I was just out of it totally.

'I was still so messed up that I used to save up my Dic and wait until night time and crush them up and inject them into my drip. But I got caught doing that.

'I remember them saying to me that they were wearing the masks because I had shingles and hepatitis, and I thought that was okay but I couldn't figure out why they had on full body-suits. They made my mother and father wear gloves and masks as well when they came in to see me and I wasn't allowed any other visitors. It was really scary.

'I was just lying there in the bed feeling very weak and thinking that when I got out I would have to seriously think about stopping taking Dic because it was really screwing me up.

'One of the nurses was very nice to me and I remember asking her why they were wearing the suits and she said she thought it was because of the hepatitis. She said certain strains of it were very infectious and that they weren't sure what I had.

'I got very sick a couple of times and I almost died. I remember having an "out of body" experience where I was up in the corner of the room looking down at my body and my parents crying and the doctor saying that if I made it through the next twenty-four hours I had a chance. And thinking: I'm fine. Here I am up in the corner of the room. There's not a bother on me.'

John had heard about AIDS. He had read about it in *Time* magazine, but it hadn't crossed his mind that it had anything to do with him.

'Then when I was a bit healthier a doctor who was good to me came in and he said: "John, I have something to tell you and there is no easy way of telling you so I'll

It was 5 February 1986.

'I just screamed, "No...I haven't...No...", and he gave me an injection and knocked me out. I woke up and I just remember sobbing my heart out. I just couldn't believe it because I knew immediately when he said it what it meant. I wasn't that stupid. I just thought it hadn't meant anything for me. This was something that happened to gay men in San Francisco. I was the first person diagnosed in Ireland with HIV, they say. I don't know if that's true or not. I must have been one of the first anyway.

'It was never talked about among junkies. Never. Not prior to 1986. I remember thinking: My life is over. I'm going to die. I just couldn't believe it. I remember lying in that bed thinking No, No, No, this is not happening. This is all a dream. I tried to convince myself that it was a dream, but it was real. And nobody had a clue what to do about it. My mother and father were just so shocked when they were told. I was devastated - twenty-seven years old and somebody tells you you've got AIDS. And that was all I heard. He might have said "You've got the AIDS virus"," but all I heard was "You've got AIDS."

'This was before the difference between HIV infection and AIDS was understood as it is today. AIDS is a syndrome, that is, a collection of diseases or conditions which point to an underlying immune deficiency. Most doctors believe the underlying cause of the condition is HIV but it is no longer believed that everyone with HIV infection will necessarily go on to get ARC [Aids Related

Complex] or AIDS. Unfortunately the percentage of those who do has risen from about 10% at my original time of diagnosis to estimates of 40% to 70% today.

'It was the most unbelievably bad shock. I was numb. I was giddy, scared and fascinated. I remember looking at my body and wondering where it was. Trying to figure out was it in my hands? Was it in my head? Was it in my balls? Was it in my legs? Then I began reading everything about AIDS I could lay my hands on and there wasn't an awful lot in Ireland.

'All the information that I got came from English publications. Eventually when I got out of hospital I contacted the Hirchfeld Centre [Dublin Gay Centre] and Gay Health Action and I was given fifteen typed pages of A4 paper telling me bits about the virus, HTLV 3 as it was called then, and about AIDS and what it meant for me, how to look after yourself, etc.

'After I began to read about it I realised I probably had full-blown AIDS. The year before I had had pneumonia and pleurisy and that often means full-blown AIDS. It was after I had been in Coolmine. I was treated as an in-patient in Baggot Street under another name. I was only in for a few days and I got over it successfully in a couple of weeks.'

John's mother remembers the phone call coming on a Saturday morning telling them to come to the hospital.

'I said to my husband they don't usually send for you on a Saturday. You know how everything comes into your head. So we went and we were seen into a little ward and there was John, a doctor - who was a terribly nice man and always treated John like a human being - a nurse and a sister. John was crying. He had had seven pints of blood. Now he had no veins so they had to use the main artery on his neck. Then the doctor said about him being HIV positive. Now it had been all in the paper about this bug in Mountjoy Jail so I said is it what they had in Mountjoy and he said "Yes". I'll always remember saying to John, "You bloody eejit, I told you so." And then I had a good cry.

'Then there was panic in the hospital. Two nurses volunteered to look after him and they were very kind. And the doctor looked after him. Nobody else. The cleaners wouldn't go in. They wouldn't deliver his meals. His father and I went up every evening and washed his dishes for the day and made him as comfortable as possible, anything non-medical we could do. We were like spacemen going in. We had to put on body-suits, shoes, gloves, masks. How must John have felt when we walked in? I think he was about seven weeks in Patrick Dun's.

'The two nurses were very good to him. And the doctor. He sent for us one day. "Will you tell John", he said, "to stop reading. He's driving me demented. He knows more about the bloody thing than I do!"'

For John the meaning of his diagnosis began to sink in. 'At the time it was still believed that it was very infectious so that is what the body-suits were about. I think I was the first case in that hospital so they went into full-scale barrier nursing. Now they said also that it was to protect me. Because of my lowered immune system they were afraid that they would bring in viruses from the outside that would affect me. There was major fear. So much so that nurses used to come down and peek at me when they thought I was asleep. I was a very strange creature at that time.

'The doctors didn't know how to react to me. They

didn't know what to say to me. I did a lot of crying. A lot of sitting quietly. There was one nurse and she tried to talk to me about what this meant for me. She was as well clued in on it as anybody on the team that was looking after me. She tried her best to help and one doctor tried to tell me what he knew about it, and as he said himself he didn't know very much at the time. It had only just begun to creep into Ireland. Very little was actually known about the virus then. It was called HTLV 3 at the time - human T-cell lymphatic virus. I remember rolling that around on my tongue, HTLV 3...AIDS... I'm a person with AIDS. My mind went screaming off and hid, because the true horror, the true scale of what that diagnosis meant didn't sink in immediately. I was on so many drugs for both my health and my addiction.

'Being told came so completely out of the blue. I was totally unprepared. There was no inkling. I hadn't been told the test was being done and been waiting for the results.'

John was numb. 'This feeling that this couldn't be happening to me. So I was in my room with the nurse outside the door and people wearing space-suits and I knew why they were wearing space-suits now. And all the plates that came into my room were left there because nobody would take them out. The bedclothing that I used was all destroyed.

'It all contributed to this feeling that I was totally unclean, that I was something horrendously dirty and untouchable. Nobody touched me without wearing gloves and all the nurses who worked with me were volunteers because they just didn't feel that they could send young student nurses in.

'I got very little information in Patrick Dun's about my

virus. All that was going through my head was that I had AIDS and I was going to die soon and how would I cope with it. And of course all my friends found out about it because they tried to visit me and with the sealed room it was obvious that there was something major wrong.

'I think the shock would have been worse if I hadn't been on all the Diconal they were giving me. It cushioned the blow.

'And it wasn't until a lady from the Eastern Health Board bustled into my room one day wearing no protection and came over and gave me a kiss that anyone touched me. That was the first human being that had touched me for six weeks. And that was brilliant. When that woman came in and told them all what they actually needed to do, things really changed. The body-suits were done away with and people cleaned my room and I began to get treated more like an ordinary patient.'

Chapter 19

SINKING IN

John was released from hospital with enough Diconal to last him a week and advice to get treatment for his drug addiction immediately.

'I was still very weak, very thin, but a hell of a lot better than I had been. I had cleared what infections I had. I was reasonably together.'

He returned to live with his parents.

'It was like I had already died. Everybody was treating me like somebody who was already dead. I remember just sitting at home and being totally and completely blank.'

He stopped using Diconal and managed to withdraw himself on the supply he had been given on leaving hospital. He used small bits of heroin but believed he had broken his heavy habit. He was back to using with his old friends but found he just wasn't able for it. He attributes that to the shock and for a while stopped all intravenous drugs and used tranquilisers only. He began taking Temgesic intramuscularly because of the continuous pain in his legs. It was prescribed at a clinic.

He began reading voraciously about AIDS. Then he had a complete nervous breakdown and was taken to St Brendan's mental hospital.

'All I remember is sitting in the house saying I can't

cope, I can't handle this and going down to the doctor saying I can't make it. I wanted to use drugs and yet I didn't want to use drugs. So he gave me a letter for St Brendan's. I don't even remember going there. I only remember it being three days later and there I was in the hospital.

'They didn't know what to do with me. They hadn't a clue. I wasn't mentally unstable. It was, if anything, reactive depression. For some reason I told everybody I knew what was wrong with me. It was the only way I knew how to cope. Sometimes you have to make allowances for my behaviour because I'm off the wall. I'm an addict. I might be a cleanish addict, but I'm an addict.

'After a couple of days St Brendan's phoned my parents and said they couldn't really help me. They said I wasn't crazy. I was afraid and had every right to be. I was petrified with fear that I was going to die. I was lost. I felt like I was drifting away from myself. That the real essential me was gone. Nobody was touching me. Nobody was near me. I began to feel like a different species of human.

'Almost everyone I know who has got the virus feels unclean, untouchable, unlovable at first. You have to begin to love yourself again before you can let anyone else love you. You know the Whitney Houston song "The Greatest Love of All"? It's a song about loving yourself. Well, that has become somewhat of an anthem among people with AIDS. It says, "The greatest love of all is happening to me, I found the greatest love of all inside of me." It's all about loving yourself and when you've got HIV infection you really need to love yourself badly. You must remember what it was like in the beginning of 1986 in Dublin, what the papers were writing, what I was reading from the English tabloids.

'It was just unbelievable. There were all these horror stories that you could get AIDS from toilet seats and cups and kissing, and stories about people being run out of their homes for having the virus, and losing their jobs. People had finally woken up to the fact that intravenous drug users were becoming infected in large numbers and there was hysteria that we would be the group that would bridge the gap between, as they said, "perverted gay men who had brought it on themselves" and the heterosexual society. There were also wild theories that it was caused by "poppers", an Amyl Nitrate-type drug that is used by gay men in clubs and which I had used myself because it gives you a big burst of energy and you can dance like crazy. Also there tended to be stories about people deliberately infecting other people. But one or two articles were beginning to point out that we could have a major problem in Dublin due to needle-sharing, particularly with younger users.'

After leaving St Brendan's, John never really stopped using, but had stopped using at the level he had been. Now that he knew he was carrying the virus in his bloodstream it was crucial that he did not share needles with other addicts. However the world of addiction is not a sane or logical place.

'I used to always have my own syringe because I used green needles, the big long ones. But sometimes people would use my barrel and on a number of occasions people actually used my works even though I told them that I had HIV infection. I knew that you could get it from needles but all I did was clean the works out as best as I

93

could. I used to really hate giving them to anybody but when you are an addict the desire to use overrides everything else. You lose all sense of reality and sense of proportion. Everybody knew what was wrong with me. I had heard that there were some people in Coolmine who had been diagnosed, but they were still out there. I was in the real world.'

The reaction of John's friends varied. Some just took it in their stride, but they were the minority. Others didn't want anything to do with him. Some wouldn't smoke a joint with him. Some people he used to know well wouldn't let him past the front door. But he was gratified to find that his long-term friends stuck by him.

His health was not good and he was plagued with rashes and thrush. He also got shingles, and alternated between bouts of diarrhoea and constipation. Around this time he began to get the headaches which have been a constant fact of life ever since. And his eyesight began to give problems. Since then he has periods of a few days at a time when his sight is badly distorted.

Then he got £8,000 in compensation for the Dorset Street motorcycle accident he had had some years earlier. He gave £3,800 to his parents and immediately began to spend the rest on heroin. That put an end to the short period of comparative abstinence.

'I remember being in a room with six people and having a fix, and all six used the works directly after me. And they knew because I had told them. They said they didn't care because they thought they had already got it. I said what about if you haven't? You definitely don't want to be as sick as I have been. But no, they needed their fix.'

After a time he wanted to quit again and became

involved in the Anna Liffey Project, a day-care project for addicts in Abbey Street. It had been set up basically to try and help inner-city addicts. 'Because I lived in Ringsend I fitted into their catchment area. But I found I couldn't relate to most of the junkies down there. Nobody else had HIV infection. I left after a few weeks. But the staff there gave me the first ever contact I had with the Terrence Higgins Trust.'

And he began going to see a psychologist who worked for a group called Cairde. 'He was the first person to ask me what did I actually know about HIV infection. He said that if I did have AIDS then I would have to come to terms with certain things. It was he who suggested that I go to England for a second diagnosis.'

To go to England John needed a report so he asked the doctor in Patrick Dun's Hospital to prepare a report for him. The doctor who had treated him there wrote to the other hospitals involved and got their notes on John, and on 19 May 1986 supplied John with a letter of introduction to the doctor in charge of the Drug Rehabilitation Unit in St Mary's Hospital in Paddington. To John's utter horror the resulting report said that he had been first diagnosed as HIV positive the previous summer in Our Lady's Hospital, Navan.

'Navan had done the test in June 1985, and they had told St Vincent's. But it wasn't until Patrick Dun's did their own test in February 1986 that I found out. I remember thinking that I had had sex with several women during that time and thinking, Oh my God, I wonder have I given it to them?

'I freaked. I knew I'd have to tell the women I had slept

95

with. It also meant that all the people I had used with from June of '85 to January of '86 all needed to be told. That was at least twenty people. I copped a responsible attitude straight away.

'That almost killed me, that knowledge. It was bad enough saying that at least I had known since February so I'm not to blame for anything beforehand. But then to think that they had actually done a test behind my back and they knew. It explained why Vincent's and Jervis Street wouldn't let me in. It explained why I had been feeling so bad. Yet nobody told me. Nobody told my family. My family were cleaning up blood after me even when I had HIV infection but we didn't know it. It left me feeling very very angry.'

John's mother is also resentful about not being told. 'When I think of the places we found needles and I picked them up. To think he may have had that virus. If we had known I might have taken more precautions. I mean, the rest of us were in the house.'

John had had girlfriends between the summer of '85 and hospitalisation. He hadn't had sex with them since December so initially he thought they were safe.

'Telling those women was so heavy. That was so fucking hard. They freaked out, and they went and had HIV tests. One of them was positive. She had been an addict so there was a possibility that she picked it up herself and that it had nothing to do with me. But not in her mind. She was sure I gave it to her. She accused me of giving it to her and not caring. It was even a possibility that I got it from her, but in her mind it was convenient to blame me. She has since died from AIDS. She continued using, moved to London and died in 1987. By the time she died she realised that we both probably already had the infection at the time anyway. She had been a prostitute and drug user since she was thirteen. It was all so chaotic.'

Now that it was clear that a HIV test was positive some time before he had been told, John contacted *Hot Press* with his story. *Hot Press* is a Dublin-based magazine that mixes music, current affairs and investigative journalism. There he met journalist Fiona Looney, who remembers him as being 'absolutely pathetic' when she first talked to him. But they took his story seriously and arranged for John to be driven to Our Lady's Hospital in Navan, where the first HIV test had been carried out during his hospitalisation there in June 1985. The hospital conceded that they had done the test and said that they had sent on the results to John's GP and to St Vincent's. This, they maintained, was normal procedure.

John was furious that they hadn't contacted him, and said so in no uncertain terms when they met the consultant. The consultant claimed that the report had been sent to John's home, and the address when checked was correct in the hospital's records. John had no recollection of receiving the letter. They could go no further and they agreed to disagree.

The *Hot Press* article, written by Fiona Looney and Audrey Gaughan, was published on 17 July 1986 under the banner headline 'I Wasn't Told I Had AIDS'. Here, John (called Frank) described himself as a biological time bomb who was returned to the community and an active sex life and continued drug abuse.

John lodged a complaint with the Department of Health regarding his treatment at Our Lady's, Navan, and St Vincent's, Dublin. The Department launched an investigation, the results of which are contained in a letter to John from the press officer of the Department, dated 17 February 1987. This letter details John's various stays in hospital in May and June of 1985 and the consultant's dissemination of the HIV positive result to the hospitals mentioned and to John's GP. John's complaint was dismissed. The Department concluded that the consultant had no knowledge of attempts made by John to contact the hospital to discuss the matter, that arrangements had been made to do this when he had, and that 'in the circumstances the consultant went to reasonable lengths to get the information to you'.

Chapter 20

DESPERATION

In summer of 1986 John headed for London. He was quite ill and was hospitalised in St Mary's in Paddington. In the absence of any opportunistic infections they diagnosed his condition as AIDS related complex, or ARC as it is usually known. He hadn't told his family where he was going. His mother was frantic.

'When John was told he was body positive he came home here and we were looking after him. Then he disappeared for five days. I was up the walls. I didn't know where he was. I tried all his friends but nobody had seen him. He had got the money together and he had flown to London and had gone to Paddington General Hospital. Unfortunately it was worse. They diagnosed ARC, AIDS related complex. He came home here and he told me it was worse.'

John was still using heroin on a sporadic basis, though he had claimed he was not in the *Hot Press* article. His life was still a complete and utter mess - 1986 was not looking very good from any perspective. Except that he was still living at home and his mother was doing what she could.

'We talked about it and that Sunday night we were sitting here, my friend and I having a cup of tea, and Avril went up the stairs and I think the road heard her screaming. He had swallowed everything in sight.'

John remembers doing it quite deliberately.

'I was lying at home and I began thinking about the situation I was in. My mother and father and sister and brothers and some friends were all downstairs and I was lying on my bed listening to my walkman. I began to ask myself why I was continuing on with this struggle. Why was I alive? I felt totally isolated. So I went downstairs and got a cup of tea, said goodnight to everybody and went upstairs and took every tablet I had. I got into bed and pulled the covers over my head. That's all I remember. And for some unknown reason my sister decided to come up and check on me and she found me just beginning to go completely out of it.'

They phoned an ambulance and got him in to St Vincent's. The hospital knew he was body positive but he received the usual emergency treatment and they managed to pump him out and save his life. It was 4 a.m. before they got the all clear, and he spent four days recovering in hospital.

His mother went up to see him next day. 'I was crying and he was crying. "I just can't take it, Ma," he said. "This is getting worse and worse." I didn't understand, so he explained to me what ARC was. He must have been feeling dreadful.'

His mother is quite convinced that John seriously intended to kill himself. 'I remember it because he came down in his underpants, and a friend and I were sitting here and I said, "John, have you no shame." He made a cup of tea and then he came down for a second cup of water and Avril said to me: "Is he all right, Mam? Is he back on drugs?" "No," I said, "He's not." And she said, "Well he's funny", and she went up the stairs.'

Avril is more sceptical. 'My Ma snapped at me when I said he was stoned out of his head. He was supposed to be off drugs at the time.

'There were about six empty bottles but I don't know how many he had taken. I think when he came down the stairs that was a cry for help. He was already stoned. He had a bottle of Coke and Lucozade up in the room if he was thirsty.

'There were two notes. One you could hardly make out at all. The other was just: "Goodbye Ma and Da. Sorry for all I put you through. Tell the kids I love them." It started off with his best writing and got worse. Before he got in the ambulance I nearly killed him because I boxed the face off him. I kept on saying, "The cheek of you."'

But John remembers differently.

'I remember when I woke up just thinking, Oh no, I'm still alive. I couldn't believe it. I was really pissed off because it had been a dead serious attempt. There had been no talking about it. It had been a decision that had been made instantly and it seemed the right thing to do so I went for it never thinking how are my family going to feel when they find me dead up here.

'I failed anyway. I had taken more than enough drugs to kill myself. I almost did, even though they got to me very quickly.

'I felt absolutely desperate - depressed, hopeless, helpless and useless. I had been using again. I just thought it was going to continue on until I died. I would just keep using. So I just thought, Why don't I die now. And I was feeling so sick. I had had enough. I couldn't go on. I had reached the end of my tether. 'And while I was in hospital two friends of mine that used to arrive over from England all the time with smack came to visit me and they brought me lots of nicknacks, including some smack. I remember smoking the smack in the hospital and thinking: Nothing has changed. I was prevented from killing myself. Now I'm doomed. I'm back into this trap of heroin addiction that I just cannot seem to get out of. I'm totally stuck.'

Chapter 21

NARCOTICS ANONYMOUS

Things continued much as before. He was soon back in Patrick Dun's Hospital again with another DVT. He was weak and the series of diarrhoea, thrush and shingles continued. He suffered excruciating headaches and continuous painssin his legs, because the circulation was so restricted. He also began to develop some spots on his legs which he didn't think anything of at the time.

'My family felt that they had failed, that somehow they had let me down. I just remember feeling: Why did you stop me? I'd be happier dead and you'd be happier. You wouldn't have to go through watching me die slowly. They were saying that they loved me. They didn't want me to die. They wanted me to live.

'I needed to talk so badly about my addiction. I had nothing to live for. There was no woman in my life. My friends were there but I felt that they didn't understand me. I felt my family were trying but we were in a hopeless situation.

'There were still always fights about money and about gambling. And there was the tension for them of never knowing whether I was using or not using. They were supportive, but it was very difficult. Niall doesn't like shouting, so they argued quietly. And there was hassle between me and Avril, and Avril and my father. But it was supportive in an odd way because all of this shit had gone on before I had the virus. So very little had changed except that I had my own toothbrush that was kept separate. If I bled at home or had soiled underwear my mother would tend to wash that separately, using bleach. We led a pretty normal life. It was as if the family closed ranks and nobody else could say anything about me, but they could say whatever they liked. My brother Patrick used to tell AIDS jokes all the time, but that was just his way of coping.

'Everybody on the road where I lived seemed to like me and have time for me, but I felt that they all knew and that they were talking about me. I felt that the family were being put through an awful lot of shit that they could do without. I felt really bitter that the suicide had been prevented. I really wanted to die even though I knew that the next year I would probably get £10,000 from the Ballsbridge motorbike accident. My life had become intensely painful, really too difficult to go on with. I had a family who loved me and who really showed they cared but I just felt so hopeless.'

John then tried Narcotics Anonymous and found that it was some help for him. NA is a worldwide network of small groups of addicts and ex-addicts who meet regularly to help each other stay off drugs. They follow a 'twelve steps to recovery' approach similar to that used by Alcoholics Anonymous or Gamblers Anonymous. John found the approach palatable. There were addicts to talk to who accepted they were addicts as he did.

'NA was like the last hope for a dying man. I clung to it. I needed it really badly. I was going to two meetings a day. I was going to the movies a lot, hanging out in coffee shops with people and trying not to take drugs. I didn't always succeed. I kept slipping up. I was still on Temgesic all the time but I didn't think of that as drugs. It was for the pain in my legs. It was from a doctor on a genuine prescription. I didn't feel I got a hit out of it. Other people will tell you they do. I think it was because my body was so used to opiates.

'What worked for me about NA was that I knew I was an addict and when you introduce yourself you say, "My name is John and I am an addict." You only use first names. For me, being able to stand up and admit that I was an addict and hear other people admit it, and talk to others about what it felt like to be an addict, even if you weren't using drugs that day, was good. Some people think if you take the drugs away that's it. But addiction is a disease. NA is based on the idea that addiction is a fatal disease. There are only three outcomes: jails, institutions, or death. I found being able to talk about problems, about my parents and so on, to "share" as they call it, was very good for me. But I found that very few people wanted to listen to what I had to say about my HIV infection. It really used to freak people out. I was their living nightmare sitting among them. They had all been on the streets using drugs and sleeping around and a lot of them hadn't had HIV tests. Some people began to say that NA was for dealing with drug addiction and not AIDS and that was when I became disillusioned. But NA does work. I still live by a lot of NA philosophy. I take every day at a time. I try not to have massive expectations and project into the future.'

In January 1987 John was busted again with a quarter of a gramme of heroin in a friend's house. He was charged with possession.

'I just thought: Oh my God, here we go again. I'm just

back in all the shit again, police on my back, a court case hanging over me.' (Because of that arrest John still cannot return to Ireland without fear of imprisonment, a risk he is not willing to take with his illness.)

Chapter 22

BORDERLINE

John had hit rock bottom and he knew it. The daily battle with drugs continued, and with some success. He was still in NA. He had not stopped using but he had cut down dramatically. He watched the media coverage on AIDS with interest, in particular the BBC TV campaign in Britain in February and the coverage on RTE Irish television during the week of 11 May 1987, when there was a major programme on the subject each night.

'There was an amazing heightened awareness in Dublin of HIV infection and the issues surrounding AIDS. I watched the Today Tonight programmes on RTE and I just thought they weren't getting across the reality of what it meant. You know, that it was real people that were involved and not these cardboard cutout pathetic junkies that were shown. Ordinary people were affected.'

On a whim, John decided to phone Aonghus McAnally, presenter of the Borderline AIDS Special programme, at RTE. I (John Masterson) was the producer of Borderline, and we were to transmit a live programme about AIDS, with particular reference to younger viewers. We intended to present the issues straightforwardly, in a way that would be real to viewers in their teens and twenties. We felt it was important to have a person with AIDS on our panel. This had never been done on RTE and we thought it was important to dispel myths about being in the same room as or touching people with AIDS. But the panellist who had agreed to appear phoned the morning of the programme to say he was too ill. Then John called. Aonghus spoke to him on the phone and then arranged to meet him. They went to Wynn's Hotel and spoke for an hour and a half. Aonghus was impressed by his story and his sincerity and invited him to come to RTE and talk further.

'I just rang because I wanted to talk to somebody about AIDS and somebody had told me that the programme was going out live, so that meant that nobody could mess around with what I said. I decided that if I could possibly do anything to stop one person getting infected then I would do whatever I could, and if that involved going public my parents agreed that it was up to me. They weren't exactly ecstatic about the thoughts of me being identified and recognised as their son, but they put up with it stoically.

'And I felt I needed to do it. That things needed to be said that weren't being said and I felt that I could probably say them. It was also important to show that this wasn't just a gay disease, because there was still a bit of that attitude. I wanted to say that addicts were suffering and that addicts were just ordinary people.

'I had given some thought to where I had picked up the virus. At the time it just seemed obvious that it was from needle-sharing. But thinking back I had had sex with so called "high risk" women in half the capitals of Europe. I could just as easily have picked up the infection sexually. It doesn't really make any difference.

'And I was more at peace with myself by then. I had

come to accept that I had ARC and I believed that I could continue on like that for quite a while. I wanted to make a difference. I wanted to stop anybody else getting infected.'

John arrived at RTE on time and seemed straight. (I later learned that he had used the day before, but not the day of the programme or the day after.) He showed me letters from various doctors and I was satisfied that he was genuine and that he was right for the programme. That was the first time I met John.

He asked that he be identified only as 'John' in order to spare his parents some little bit. We also arranged that after Borderline, he would join the panel on a radio show which was due to run an AIDS phone-in until 2 a.m.

John's performance on Borderline was remarkable and won widespread praise. He talked about how ill he had been and how careful he was of his health now. He described his time in hospital. He epitomised the responsible attitude and argued for safe sex, criticising the government campaign for focussing more on the dangers of casual sex than on the need for safe sex - this seemed to be influenced more by Catholic moral teaching than by the problem that was to be addressed. He attacked the narrowmindedness of chemists who would not sell condoms. He called for a needle-exchange policy and a Methadone maintenance programme, pointing out that this had been successful in Amsterdam. He believed that if longterm Methadone maintenance was available, rather than short detoxification programmes, that many more addicts would be able to come off street drugs. He emphasised that AIDS could happen to any person. It wasn't just freaks. No one's parents thought it could happen to their child. But it could.

'After the programme I felt bare, after the radio especially. These were real people ringing up. I felt a little bit proud but very scared, wondering what this was going to mean for me and my family. Up to that point nobody had gone public in Ireland. As far as I know there was nobody who was willing to stand up and say: Yes, I've got ARC, or, I've got AIDS.

'And, Yes, there was ego involved. There was the feeling that this will once again differentiate me from the masses. What other chance would I ever have of being interesting enough to be on television? And yet that wasn't the overriding reason I did it. The overriding reason was because I wanted to stop even one other person getting infected if I possibly could.

'But I must admit I enjoyed it. It was quite flattering for people to want to know your opinions. My ego lapped it up but I always tried to keep in mind the reasons why I was doing it.

'My parents were very proud of me. They said I did very well and most of my friends were quite pleased but said that it was a very big step. Some thought I was foolish and that I should have thought of my parents more. Some people just turned away from me. They didn't want to be seen with me in case people thought they had AIDS. Most of the reaction was positive. Even the people on the road I lived on all came out and said, "Well done."'

His mother was pleased with the reaction too. 'Believe it or not, people were very, very sympathetic. They were saying, "How do you cope?" That kind of thing. Nobody has ever made a nasty remark.

110

'Though there was one incident with a friend and her kids. Oh God, I felt for him. She said goodbye to John and she kissed him and I said, "Give John a kiss," to the kids. "Come on," she said. "We're in a hurry." I was hoping John didn't notice. But he did.'

Avril hated the publicity. 'I didn't want everybody to know. I couldn't cope with it being in the papers. I was down at my friend's one day and my Ma rang to say John was going on Borderline. She said they wanted to make sure everybody agreed. I said: "Please ask him not to. I don't want everybody knowing our business." But he still just went ahead. She never said it to him. That's when I gave up my job. I never went back there. I couldn't go back to face them, knowing that they knew. Where I work now nobody knows.

'Maybe now I can see some of the good points but I still don't forgive him for going on Borderline. I didn't watch it until four weeks later. People said to me he was very good but I told them I didn't watch it.'

In retrospect, John believes it was the right thing to do. 'It was necessary for me to do it. It did some good. I think that was a worthwhile programme. It said a lot about the state of awareness about HIV and AIDS in Ireland at the time.'

John's resolve to completely quit drugs was strengthening around this time. 'It was like a dawning realisation that no longer did using take care of the pain of my existence. I had always used drugs to keeps down feelings and pain, the pain of difference, of strangeness, or uniqueness, the pain of life. And it just didn't work any more.

'Drugs and AIDS had begun to alter the priorities in my life. My HIV infection had brought about a sort of

111

spiritual reassessment of what was going on in my life. A lot of that came from some of the psychologists I had talked to. I was beginning to achieve some personal growth, just a little bit. Just enough to begin questioning where I was and trying to look for a way out and a way forward rather than just staying in the shit I was in. I had a voice in my head that was saying, Move or die.

'I had seen a different way of life by going to NA. I had seen that it was possible for an addict to accept that he was an addict and yet get on and live a clean life. For the first time I saw addicts recovering and I believed that it was possible for me to recover even though I had AIDS related complex as well.'

Chapter 23

CHINA

The compensation for John's second motorcycle accident was finally paid. It amounted to just under £10,000. He gave his parents half of it to build a dormer room in the house and he immediately booked a holiday in China for himself. He went to London, and the following day flew with his tour group to Peking. What was intended as the holiday of a lifetime turned into yet another nightmare.

'I was going on my own and I got introduced at the airport to the guy I would be sharing with. He was a doctor and I thought, Just my luck!

'The first evening we were allowed to go off around Peking. So I went down to a People's Market. It was marvellous. People everywhere, smiling and talking and milling around. I bought a few souvenirs. It was brilliant. I went to a performance at an ordinary people's theatre. When I came out people were looking at me and some of them touched me because foreigners are still strange there. It was a great night. Eating strange food and just soaking up the atmosphere. I had been told that one of the greatest sights is to look out your window at six o'clock in the morning, which I did. All you see is bicycles on these big broad streets. And the silence is awesome, because all you can hear is the whishing of the tyres with the odd car honking now and then.

'We got up early the next morning and drove out to the Ming tombs. The Ming tombs are a complex of tombs outside Peking where the Ming emperors were buried. They have excavated some of the tombs and you can go into one of them where they have all the funeral items, including these jade masks and full jade figures. All along the entrance there is the giant triumphal walkway with statues of heavenly beasts and gods and demons to protect the tombs. It really is an awesome sight. I'd never seen anything like it.

'There were twenty-two of us in the tour party and everyone was very excited about it because it was a great holiday. We had lunch and then went on to the Great Wall of China. We all split up to walk along the Wall. It was breathtaking. You'd have to see it to understand the scale of it. It's gigantic.

'Then, as I was climbing one of the watchtowers a woman in front fell and hit me and knocked me off the steps. My back was hurt so I got carried down and they put me on the bus and we were taken back to the hotel. I was in quite a lot of pain but I could shuffle along in between two people. On the way we stopped at a clinic. It was one of these hotel clinics for a huge block of apartments. There was a woman doctor and she wanted to use acupuncture on me. So I told her she couldn't and being responsible I told her why. I told her about the HIV infection and hepatitis. So she said Okay, through the interpreter, and that was it.

'My back was still sore but bearable and that night we went to the Peking Opera. At the intermission our tour guide came along with these three Chinese people in suits - most Chinese didn't wear suits. The guide asked how my back was and offered to take me to a hospital so

I was happy enough about that. They said I should come with them because they wanted to make sure I was okay and to examine me for insurance purposes. The doctor that I was sharing with offered to come too.

'They drove us past the State Foreigners' Hospital. I could see the sign, but they continued on down the road to another hospital that looked like a prison. It was a big square building with bars on the windows. It turned out to be an infectious disease control hospital.

'We were brought in and the English doctor who had come with me was taken to one room with the Chinese officials and interpreter and I was taken to another across the corridor. The door was left ajar and I could hear them talking.

'I left the room and walked down the corridor and all the rooms had bolts on the outside which I thought was strange in a hospital. The only place I had seen that was St Brendan's. I looked in and in one room there was a man who was covered in sores and his face just seemed to be gone. Another person was all purple and yellow and was just lying in a bed sweating and shivering. A couple of other people were just lying under the covers moaning. I thought, Holy fuck, what is this place? I freaked out. So I ran back to the room and shouted "What's happening?" at them. A couple of the Chinese orderlies grabbed me and physically propelled me into the room. They stood at the door and I was never allowed out of their sight.

'Then the medical people came over from the other room and said to calm down and they talked a little and then they said, "You have AIDS." So I said I hadn't and that I had AIDS related complex. "You have AIDS. You cannot stay in our country. You shouldn't have been let in." And I just kept on saying that I had ARC but not AIDS.

'So then they said they needed to do a blood test. And they kept on asking me was I the doctor's lover. The doctor was very upset at this and began crying. He said things were getting very heavy and he didn't want to be involved. I knew then that things weren't going to go well. He was very freaked out. I don't know what they had said to him. I told them I wasn't gay and I explained that we had never met before the airport where we were introduced and told we would be sharing.

'So I asked for the Irish consul and said I wanted to go back to the hotel. But they said I must give a blood sample first. I kept on refusing. I just didn't want to. I felt they were invading my privacy and I had admitted I was HIV positive so there was no point. So they said they were going to take a sample and I still refused to do it voluntarily. So four of them grabbed me and held me in a chair with one of them sitting on my legs and they couldn't get a vein so they slit my arm and they held a bottle underneath to collect the blood. All four of them in body-suits.

'It was so primitive. They didn't even have antiseptics. They were using iodine and bits of cotton wool wrapped around little wooden sticks. I became hysterical and started screaming and thrashing around. I thought they were going to keep me. You know, this is China. They're going to keep me like this.

'Then they left me alone and I was just sobbing my heart out. I couldn't believe what was going on. A few hours later they came back and said they were taking me back to the hotel but that I would have to stay in my room. So I said Yes - anything to get back to the hotel.

116

The Director of the hospital told me that they were petrified of the public health implications of AIDS getting loose in the general population. I told them I was responsible about my illness, but it didn't make any difference.

'Back at the hotel I was met by the tour guide and the representative of the travel company. They weren't even allowed talk to me. I was just told to go straight to my room. The doctor who was sharing with me had asked for another room. I took some sleeping tablets but I couldn't go to sleep. I was too freaked out. I just felt like I had been raped. I looked outside in the middle of the night and there was an armed guard outside and he told me to go back in.

'In the morning a guy called Brendan Ward who was a Third Secretary in the Irish embassy arrived. He seemed a nice enough man and he came up to my room. The Chinese had said I had to stay in my room but they hadn't said anything about the rest of my holiday. I was feeling really bad, and Brendan Ward said he would get the details and try and sort it out. He came back after about an hour or so to tell me that they wanted me to leave the country. I said I had paid for the holiday and I wanted to have it. He said he didn't think they were going to let me. He told me that they had brought in a law on May 1st that said that nobody who is known to be HIV positive could be admitted to China.

'So he went off again to see if anything could be done. I just felt like a caged animal. I was in a strange country thousands of miles from home. I had been honest. I had told them what was wrong with me. And my honesty had got me locked up in a hotel room. 'After a few hours Brendan Ward came back and he said: "John, there is no way that the Chinese are going to let you stay here. They are going to put you out on the first available plane. I'm sorry. We've tried everything at the embassy but there is nothing we can do. The Chinese are adamant, and it is their country."

'He said he would be back when it was time for me to go. So I was left in that fucking hotel room staring out over Peking thinking have I not suffered enough already. Do I need to go through this as well?

'At about seven in the evening Brendan returned and said I should pack. I had to leave. I was given some Valium and the interpreter gave me some Chinese anti-depressants. I was driven up to Tien Min Square in a government car, myself, Brendan Ward and two Chinese secret service men. They showed me The Great Hall of the People and then drove me to the airport. The airport was deserted. Brendan Ward and I sat and had a Coke. He said he was really sorry. He was magic.

'There was nobody there apart from one Chinese official standing where you walked to get on to the plane. He wouldn't take my money to pay for my exit stamp. I figured everyone else was on the plane before me. Then I was put me on an aeroplane by myself. Just the crew and me. No passengers. Then I thought I had got on first, but they shut the door. The crew put me in the first-class compartment and they sealed it. They didn't come near me. They pulled bamboo curtains around. This Chinese inspirational film came on the video screen all about exhorting the people to produce more. The bar was there open and I just drank myself into oblivion. I shouted for some food and they slid a tray of crackers and cheese under.

'Have you any idea what it feels like to be rejected by

a whole country? I felt so dirty and unclean. One of the people on the tour got in touch with me back in England and told me that when I left the hotel they took everything out of my room and burned it.'

After short stops in the United Arab Emirates and Zurich, John was back in London. British immigration people came on to the plane and checked his passport and he was allowed off the plane. It was late and he went to stay with some friends and slept for thirty-six hours. He woke up to the familiar pain of a DVT. He had a fever and thrush and shingles, all of which had come on in thirty-six hours. He was admitted to North Middlesex Hospital.

Chapter 24

FRONTLINERS

While recuperating in the North Middlesex Hospital, John made the decision to stay in England. He was aware that he needed to change the way he had been living and knew that that would be well-nigh impossible for him in Dublin. He needed to get away from the environment in which he had been using drugs for such a long time.

He spent two weeks in hospital and then went back to stay with a friend who put him up for a few weeks. It was a small flat and it was not feasible to stay there for any length of time. But he was soon to get sick again with a battery of the same recurrent problems and this time was admitted to St Mary's in Paddington.

John's expulsion from China so soon after he had become nationally known for his Borderline appearance was front-page news in Ireland. He was filmed in hospital with his parents by a Today Tonight RTE television crew.

'Everything was just crazy. I felt my life was unravelling. It was becoming a sort of absurdist play in which I had no idea what was going on. My life was out of control or so it seemed to me. Things were just happening to me rather than me planning anything. Life was just being done to me rather than me doing anything to life.'

While a patient there he tried to commit suicide again.

'I had just had enough. This time I did it by slashing my wrists in the hospital bed. Again I nearly succeeded, but as I was in a hospital I should have known they would find me. I don't know what I was thinking about. I just wanted to die. The rejection by China, the feelings that that brought back to me of uncleanness, of being dirty, of feeling like not part of the human race any more. I was out of it emotionally, physically, every which way, distraught. I just didn't know what to do, but all through that I had decided that I was going to change my life, that I wasn't going to use again.'

John signed on the English dole, which was easy to do, and decided to go on a Methadone maintenance programme. Methadone stops the physical symptoms of withdrawal. It was the breathing space he needed to stabilise himself if he was to have any hope of building a new life and Methadone was available in England on long-term prescription. John was certain that there was no way he could clean up on the two-week programmes available in Dublin. He needed a few months on 'script' to get his life in order.

'My lifestyle and my life expectation had been altered by my HIV status and now I had a chance in London to make a new start. I had no idea what shape that life would take. And after all the brouhaha about China I didn't want to go home and face all the attention. I felt that I could achieve things in England that I couldn't achieve in Ireland. I didn't know what services were available but I had heard that there were more services available for people like me.'

And crucially, there existed a warrant for his arrest in Dublin, so that John could not safely return home. While he was ill his court case for heroin possession came up.

His doctor wrote to the court on 18 June 1987 saying that he was unfit to travel. A bench warrant was issued for John's arrest when he did not appear. The Garda Press Office points out that as the charge John faced was a felony, the judge had no option but to issue a warrant for his arrest. It was not a discretionary matter.

In London, John got in touch with the Terrence Higgins Trust, which is a charitable trust that was set up and named after one of the first people to die of AIDS in England. Its function is to provide information on HIV infection and AIDS and to provide and monitor services for people with the infection. As well as producing educational literature they run a telephone helpline and also provide a counselling service. The Terrence Higgins Trust sent along a counsellor to talk to him. He was invited into their office and met someone else with AIDS for the first time.

His name was Ron McEvoy and meeting him was one of the changing points in my life. He has since passed away and I miss him dearly. I had met nobody who was sick like me and it was a joy. It was an unmitigated pleasure to just talk to somebody who knew what I was feeling, who I didn't have to explain my feelings of self doubt, of self revulsion, to. And this one person showed me in a couple of hours of talking that it was possible to live with all of these feelings and live a reasonably good life. He introduced me to Frontliners of which he was the leader. It was Ron who first told me that the purpose of Frontliners and of all those with AIDS should be to enable people with AIDS and HIV infection to live as powerfully and as long as possible. Life with dignity.

'Coming from Dublin where all the people I had met with HIV infection were addicts and straight, it was quite a culture shock suddenly meeting all gay men - not most of them, everybody. But I didn't care. They were human beings. I've never been homophobic so it didn't bother me that they were gay men. That was the way the disease had infected people over here. But they understood what I was feeling. They knew really deep down what it was like to be ill with AIDS and to be discriminated against. They were outsiders just like me. They belonged to another élite, the little club of gay men, and yet they had banded together for strength and they were a community. And I'd never had a community since my hippie days. Addict life had been pretty much for yourself, by yourself.

'My feeling on entering the Terrence Higgins Trust and meeting people with AIDS was a great sense of relief, a feeling that I belonged immediately. It never crossed my mind that there would be a place for me, but I knew that I wanted to work with people with AIDS. I needed counselling, which I got immediately. I was counselled by a professional counsellor and also by Frontliners. The counselling was brilliant. It involved sitting me down and saying, John, do you know what having ARC means for you? It involved sitting down with other people who had the infection and asking them how they were surviving day-to-day. Then we went right back to my diagnosis, making me relive it and talk about the feelings that came up and about how I was treated in Dublin, and about the fear that I had had to deal with.

'Also I got involved in a self-help group for HIV infected addicts that I helped to set up in the Terrence Higgins Trust. We used to meet every Friday night with a professional facilitator and we could discuss problems that we were having with our addiction and with our infection. It got to be a very close group where a lot of people did a lot of growing. It was very important for me to sit there and talk with other straight addicts. Just as gay men have great empathy with each other so have addicts. Addicts can really be of great help to each other. There is a great sense of identification when you don't have to keep explaining things to people. They understand on a very deep level what you are going through. It is the reason why Narcotics Anonymous works as well. So we are setting up a support group called Mainliners for addicts with HIV to provide that service.

'And I got involved with Frontliners which is made up of people with AIDS or ARC. They wanted me to join them because they felt that I could be a useful and beneficial member, that I had a lot to offer because of my experience of addiction, but that I also could gain a lot by being involved in the group.

'It was a big step for me meeting those people and getting unconditional love. I had only ever had unconditional love when I was in Narcotics Anonymous. This now was love that accepted that I had ARC. They told me that they loved me and that I was an okay person and that it was all right to be me and that my feelings were my own. Stuff I really needed to hear.

'At this stage I had just fully accepted from the bottom of my soul that I had HIV infection, that I had ARC, and that there was nothing I could do about it. All I could do was try and live as positively as I could. All the wishing and the railing and ranting in the world would not change the fact that I had ARC.'

Chapter 25

THE AIDS MASTERY

Soon after joining Frontliners, John heard about an intensive self-development session known as the AIDS Mastery, run by Sally Fisher, a therapist from New York.

'The AIDS Mastery was a turning point for me. It was a weekend about getting in contact with your feelings. It was about getting deep down and opening up to other people, which I had just begun to do with Frontliners, but the AIDS Mastery showed me that it was possible to do it with anybody in the proper environment and where people understood.

'The make-up of the weekend was eighteen professionals, four people with AIDS and fifty helpers, so there were about seventy people there. It was set up by Sally Fisher and run by the Actor's Institute in London. It is a thing that has been run in New York for a number of years and is run all over America now. Sally comes over to London to lead them herself occasionally, and I was very lucky to be on one when she was there. And I stood up in front of those seventy people and I told them that I felt like shit, that I felt really dirty and unclean, that I had immense problems coming to terms with the fact that I had ARC, that I had been ill, that I had been given Extreme Unction when I had been sick the first time in Patrick Dun's.

'There was a part of me at that time back in Patrick Dun's that wanted to live, because it would have been so easy just to surrender to death. And the suicide attempts, in retrospect, seemed to have been occasions when I became overwhelmed by all the bad things about being a person with AIDS.

'So at the AIDS Mastery I stood in front of all these people and I cried openly, and I just cried and cried and cried because there was so much sadness inside me. And then, miraculously, by all these affirmations and people telling me that I was good and that I was deserving of love and deserving of care and that I was a unique human being, I slowly began to accept myself on a really deep level, to accept myself as an addict, to accept myself as a person with AIDS related complex. It was a time for me to grieve about everything and to come through the grief. There was acceptance at the end of the grief. There was almost forgiveness of myself. Almost saying: You didn't do this to yourself. This happened. The lifestyle you led put you at risk, but when you were leading that life you didn't know. So I forgave myself. I'm not to blame. I'm ultimately responsible, but not in a blameworthy sort of way.

'The purpose of the weekend was for everybody involved with AIDS - those of us living with AIDS, those who loved people with AIDS and who worked with people with AIDS - to be in contact with our own feelings in an intimate, personal and immediate way. It was so that those of us with the disease could begin living powerfully with AIDS.

'The Mastery was absolutely essential to my personal development and it opened up the possibility that I could really begin helping people. My personality had

had a sabbatical. It was almost like I had stopped developing at about age seventeen and I suddenly had an awful lot of growing up to do. I felt very young. I noticed that I wasn't very good at ordinary living. I had no living skills. I needed a course in remedial housekeeping because I had no idea how to keep myself clean, keep my clothes clean, keep the house clean. I had never done it. I had no experience of shopping. I had no experience of keeping a budget together.

'Also with people I only had two sorts of relationships. Either you were my friend and I loved you and you counted in my life or you were somebody else - and everybody else was there to be used, usually to get drugs. Family and friends you don't rip off. It meant that I had a sort of schizoid attitude towards people. My interpersonal relations with people were really screwed up. It took me a while to realise that I could have different levels of relationships with people. Now it is wider. There are people I work with in the office, people I go for dinner with, people I can have professional relationships with.

'There was a feeling that I had come out of a long dark tunnel and it had taken the double blow of ARC diagnosis and deportation from China to break through and to really put me in contact with how I was feeling for the first time in ten years. I actually felt pain, joy, sadness, anger, and all I had felt was just numbness and revulsion. And when I accepted that I had this revulsion and sadness inside me I was also able to accept that I was capable of the opposite, of love, of caring, of being a responsible person.

'I had made the decision when I did the Borderline programme that I would do anything that I could do to stop others getting this disease. So after the AIDS Mastery I decided I was going to get involved in Frontliners in a big way. I began to work full-time in the office. At the start I made the tea, answered the phone, cleaned the office, just general dogsbody stuff that everybody did. And slowly as I got more counselling and from talking to people, they realised that I had a lot to say and that I was quite good at communicating my ideas.

'They began asking me to speak to people and to begin educating people within the Terrence Higgins Trust and Frontliners about the issues relevant to drug users. The Trust had been an almost completely gay organisation and I was one of the first heterosexual addicts with ARC or AIDS to come into contact with them who wasn't homophobic and wasn't freaked out by the fact that it was perceived as a gay organisation.

'I used to be very anti-authoritarian and now I find myself sitting on committees working with what I see as the establishment to try and get services for what I see as my people, HIV infected people. Specifically I have an interest in other addicts because I still believe that addicts get treated worse than anyone else with HIV. Addicts still don't get on the drug trials because they are thought to be unreliable. A lot of addicts aren't told they are HIV positive because doctors feel that they can't be trusted with this knowledge, that if you tell them they will go out and use more drugs and become totally off-the-wall. People are still afraid of addicts. People mistrust addicts. Every doctor has had a bad experience with an addict. When they come into a room they see an *addict* in the bed. Not a human being with problems - and with one of the biggest problems you can have - but an addict, and they think: What is this addict going to try and manipulate out of me today?

'All this involvement has been terrific for me. I began to blossom. That's the only way to put it. I began to see that I could get up every day and go into an office and work there for five or six hours, come home and make sure I ate properly, look after my health, collect my "script" every day and go to the hospital twice a week.'

John was still troubled with headaches and a kind of blindness. He was also put on a drug called Warfarin which prevents blood from coagulating and has controlled his DVTs. Between 1985 and 1987 he had been hospitalised nine times for deep venous thrombosis. He expects to be on Warfarin for the rest of his life.

'They wouldn't give me Warfarin in Dublin because no one was willing to take blood from me. Over here they have set up a different system where they only have to prick your finger to test your blood. It shows the difference between here and Ireland, that they were willing to do something quite difficult for me over here.

'By trying to live a positive way I was coming to love myself and accept myself and to care about other people. At the start I tried to keep my emotions away and not get friendly with any of the other Frontliners in case somebody would die on me. But then I let my guard down, because it was impossible to be around that much love and caring and not be a loving, caring person yourself. It has led to some real heartbreak. I've had three people die on me. It is really hard to accept people you cared about dying from a disease that you have.

'You have periods of health and periods of unhealthiness but basically you are constantly aware of your own mortality, aware that your body is infected with a virus that at any moment might turn on you and begin killing you. You see the virus turn on your friends and kill them. One friend died very slowly and very horribly. He went through everything ... Pneumocystis pneumonia, Kaposi's sarcoma, cytomegalovirus, toxoplasmosis ... he went from a lively vibrant person to a wreck. And then there was another friend who I saw on a Tuesday. He was perfectly healthy and bouncy and he died on Sunday. Those are the extremes that AIDS can take.

'It brings up fear and anger that young people in the prime of their lives are dying from a disease that nobody can do much about. Anger towards the medical profession they because they seemed to be failing. I had been used to going into hospitals and being treated and being fixed. And that doesn't seem to happen with AIDS. My experience now, having been around a lot of people with AIDS, is that it is a totally unpredictable condition. Most people only get better for a while.'

Chapter 26

AIDS - FULL-BLOWN

Around this time when all was going well, John began to develop some lesions on his legs. He had had two lesions in Dublin which had been biopsied in St James's Hospital, but he had never got the results. He asked at the hospital in London what the lesions were, the great fear being that they were Kaposi's sarcoma which is one of the conditions indicative of full-blown AIDS. They biopsied two of the new lesions and the results showed that they were non-specific melanomas, a type of non-malignant skin cancer. John was relieved that the diagnosis of his condition was still ARC.

'Then one day a few weeks later I was in the Middlesex Hospital with my file and I looked through it and I found two letters, one from St Mary's in London and it read: "As you can see from the enclosed summary, he was recently diagnosed as having Kaposi's sarcoma. I have not revealed this diagnosis to him while awaiting confirmation by our own histologists." And that was signed by the doctor in St Mary's. What had happened was that they had contacted Dublin, and St James's had told them that the things they had biopsied were Kaposi's sarcoma. And they had sent over the slides, but the slides had got lost.

'It was like a hammer-blow in the stomach. I knew that

that meant AIDS. I went back to the office and just cried and cried. I remember screaming at the doctor two days later, "Why didn't you tell me?" And he said it was because they weren't able to confirm it themselves so they didn't want to say. I said I thought I should have been told and he agreed in retrospect that I should have been but said that at the time I was very emotionally unstable so they had decided to wait until they had diagnosed it themselves.'

John remembers that day as one of the worst. 'It was not unexpected but it was still a blow. It meant having to face up to the fact that I probably didn't have a lot of years left. The reprieve felt over, because by this time I knew almost everything about the disease and its patterns so I was well aware that Kaposi's sarcoma was one of the main definitions of full-blown AIDS.'

He rang his mother to tell her.

'I was sitting here and he rang and said, "I've a bit of bad news for you, Ma." He had been waiting for the result of something on his leg, but another blotch came out and they did the test in England. It was Kaposi's sarcoma. "I won't talk now, John," I said. "Give me time to adjust." I waited about two days before we talked and I went to my own doctor in the meantime and he explained that it was one of the things that goes with full-blown AIDS. He asked me was I prepared for what would happen. I suppose I'm as prepared as I'll ever be.

'Then I decided to go over to see him. When I heard full-blown AIDS, I thought he was going to die immediately. But he looked great when I got there, but he wouldn't discuss what I should do if anything should happen to him.'

For John it put everything in very sharp focus.

'It meant that I really made the final commitment to let go of any ideas of doing anything other than working for Frontliners. A lot of what I was doing by then was going out and talking to various groups about what it is like to be an addict with AIDS ... talking to support groups, addicts, gay men, talking to nurses and doctors and home helps and the general public. This work was meaningful. It was essential, and it could help save lives. We try to disseminate the truth to go against all the misinformation that is pumped out by the English tabloid scandal sheets. People's attitude in London towards people with AIDS is quite good but it is not quite so good everywhere else in England. And Scotland is as bad as Ireland.

'By this time I had been put on benefit and I had been given a small granny-flat by Haringey Council. Later I moved to where I am now, which is a specialist housing association that was set up as a place for people with HIV infection because housing was identified as one of the most pressing needs. I applied for one and lo and behold I got the interview and I got the flat. The rent is paid by the Department of Health and Social Security. It is furnished, has all mod cons and it is mine. It is like my little refuge from the world. Everything essential for living was in this flat, including a special phone which is a "lifeline" telephone. It allows you to operate the phone remotely, and by pressing an emergency button which you carry around with you you can ring the emergency services or one of three emergency numbers that you have programmed into the memory. They know who is calling, know all your details, who your doctor is, what medicines you are on, and they get an ambulance. It is brilliant for someone like me who suffers from fits. It is exactly what it calls itself. It is a lifeline. And the rental charge is paid by the borough so you only pay for your calls.

'Coming in contact with the Terrence Higgins Trust enabled me to get all the benefits I am entitled to. Up until the benefit change in April '88 people with AIDS could get up to £100 a week. I get £82. The budget also means that I now have to pay 20% of my rates and all my water rates. I have a bus and tube pass, and a taxi card that enables me to pay £1 for a taxi costing up to £7.50 in the metropolitan area. The reason that I qualify for all these benefits is that as well as having AIDS I have such bad problems with my legs that I am registered as disabled. I can't walk very far without a lot of pain. I have a medical card which means that all medical treatment is free. I was born over here so I'm not sure if it would be the same for other Irish people. And there are a lot of charities here that give money to people with AIDS to help with bills. I don't worry about my bills. I know that if I can't pay them somebody will.

'And the Terrence Higgins Trust have provided me with a "buddy" - somebody who comes in and helps with the chores and is a friend. I can go and work in the Frontliners' office but that is mental work, answering phones, talking to people, writing letters. It is not physically tiring. At home I need help with things like the ironing, and heavy washing, or the shopping which I can't carry. But the buddy relationship is one that builds up. It is a friend. And I also go to a weekly social and meet a load of people with AIDS, people from all walks of life.

'I have an illness and I do everything I can to heal myself. At the moment I'm on Warfarin for my blood,

Methadone maintenance, Chlorpromazine, which is a tranquiliser, Epilen which is an anti-epilepsy medicine and I hope to begin on AZT again. I tried it once and I became anaemic. All the different medicines I take are necessary to keep me alive.

'I feel a lot better. I still have dreadful headaches. I still have problems with my sight. I have fits which started last November. I've had brain scans and cat scans and EEGs, and there is a slight abnormality in my brain, but nothing that would account for the type of fits I have been having. So they think it is epilepsy of some description. I keep getting rashes, thrush and herpes, all sort of minor things, bladder and bowel infections, skin infections, mouth ulcers - all stuff associated with having a compromised immune system. I've only been healthy fully about twice in the last year. Illness is a constant factor but I try not to let it overwhelm my zest for living and the pleasure I get in what I do. A lot of what I do instils a feeling of self respect in me. The feeling that I am making a difference.'

Chapter 27

ACCELERATED INNER DEVELOPMENT SYNDROME

Attitude is, John believes, the most important weapon in his personal fight against AIDS. And recently a new relationship with a woman has been a crucial help.

'It was something I had almost given up on because of the problems associated with sex between an infected and an uninfected person. My girlfriend is an ex-addict but she has been tested and she doesn't have HIV antibodies. The relationship is just like anybody else's relationship, I suppose, but there are the physical realities of safer sex, which involves always using condoms for any penetrative act. That doesn't mean that you can't express yourself sexually. It just involves a small amount of care and a bit of preparation but we're working at it together.

'I don't know where the relationship is going to go. We're only at the start. We met on an AIDS awareness training day that was put on by her at a London Polytechnic that she attends and we just hit it off immediately. And we became friends and eventually lovers.

'It has allowed me to feel even more able to feel good about myself because somebody is actually accepting me as a physical feeling caring human being as well as just on an emotional level. It is good for the ego, good for the soul, good for the body and it is good for the mind. I had forgotten how much I missed being touched in a sexual way. I was getting a lot of hugs but it is not the same. Sex is like a positive affirmation of life. It sort of says: We're really here; we're really functioning and living.

'It wasn't a snap decision, but relationships are like that. They tend to happen in spite of obstacles. My HIV is something of which we have to be constantly aware. A woman going into a relationship with me has to be aware that if she decides to have children with me, both she and the child run the risk of getting the infection themselves.

'It will last as long as we are attracted to each other and need to be with each other. There are pressures on us. The pressures of not being able to have "normal" sex. There is the question, What will her friends and her family think? There are all the difficulties around who do you tell or not tell. And how are other people going to react? And how are their reactions going to influence our reactions to each other? It is too early yet to know how complicated this can get, but I would say it could be very complicated and very emotionally draining on both of us. It will need a large amount of commitment on both sides to keep this relationship going and stable. I think because of the investment that she and I have had to make in this that it will last quite a while.

'But she is going to have to live with the constant fear that I am going to get sick. I'm sure she is going to worry even though she is going to try not to. Every little cold, every little cough, every new abscess, every new skin rash will be just as fearful for her as it is for me. We can just love each other while we can because I don't know how long I am going to be here. I haven't really got a lot of time to waste.

'It is nice to have somebody to lie next to at night and tell the problems of the day to. The job I do has quite a lot of pressure in it. I'm dealing with newly diagnosed people, people with housing and welfare difficulties. And then dealing with the death of friends all the time. People getting sick and then attending another funeral. I've been to too many funerals already, but I shall keep attending them because people are going to keep dying and probably some day people will be attending my funeral and I hope that if and when I do die this last year and however much longer I have, will in some way make up for the ten lost years, fifteen nearly, of my addiction. Because this is about the happiest I have been since I was a kid. All the struggle to get this far has been worth it.

'Now I hope to take the next step which is to get off my maintenance and become clean, drug-free, at least from mood-altering drugs. I'll never be free of drugs. I know that. But I would like to be free of heroin and all its derivatives and substitutes, and Methadone is a substitute for heroin. In the last six months I have halved my daily intake of Methadone. I take 25ml morning and evening and I'm working to get it down further. It is getting easier. I don't have the craving now to go out and use heroin. It is receding into the background and becoming less a part of my life. But I would never say that it could never happen again.

'What is uppermost in my mind now is getting stuck into the work - talking to people and trying to change attitudes. And keeping my relationship going as well. And just living, being, for as long as I possibly can. I now know that it is possible to live for quite a long time with a diagnosis of AIDS. I have friends who are alive five and six years. Sometimes it comes along and debilitates you but you keep recovering. And AZT is there now to try and halt the process. And there are other drugs in the pipeline. Nobody knows what might happen in five years. If I am still alive we could be looking at at least a treatment situation. They might be able to slow it down the way AZT hopes to. So we live in hope.

'Until then I do everything I can. I use positive imagery, massage, counselling. I take multi-vitamins in the morning, and zinc and silenium. Everything to help me cope with the reality of my life. I use a couple of alternative therapies as well, holistic medicine treating the whole body. I use the therapeutic power of colours. And an Eastern treatment called Reichi which is a Tibetan energy therapy. I really find it very good. A lot of people in America use it and it is just beginning to take off over here.

'Right at the moment life is good. It is unrecognisable from what it was two years ago. It is amazing what a difference even a year makes. But the diagnosis of AIDS also made a difference. It put everything in sharp focus.

'I know I should try and enjoy the rest of my life. It might be long or it might be short, but how I live it is what is important. Not how long, but how well. And I have been healthier in the last few months than I have been since 1984. I don't ever expect to run a marathon, but I would expect to start jogging again, and swimming. As long as my Kaposi doesn't start somewhere else on my body.'

On her recent visit to London, John's mother discussed death with him for the first time. 'He's giving leaflets to people and I read them, so I said to him that he would want to practise what he preached. You're telling people to get their affairs in order. He said, "I have nothing to leave, Mam." So I took the ball on the hop and asked him what did he want me to do if anything happened to him. "I was waiting on that," he said, "but I didn't want to broach the subject with you." He said he had lovely friends in England and he wanted us to come over and have a cremation service. It is a terrible thing to have to discuss. So I asked him what to do with his bits and pieces and he said I could have them. He asked if I had the money to come over and I told him I had it put away. And the only other thing he wants is to come home but he can't. I've been in contact with the Guards and they won't drop the charge. They want his cooperation, but with the kind of people he was dealing with his life wouldn't be worth living. John never hurt anybody only himself and his family.'

Dealing with death is difficult for John. 'When my mother talks about me not talking to her about my possible death I think that was because I really didn't know how to approach it at the time. I hadn't really thought about it enough myself. It wasn't until a few people close to me died that it really struck me. I remembered how close I had been to death. I really began to question how I felt about my death. Not death as an abstract concept, but my physical death. There has been a change in the last few years and I don't feel that this life is all that there is. There is a growing certainty in me that there is something after death. I have a feeling inside me that there is a lot more to come, a belief that things will work out. I really did survive a lot and there is a part of me that thinks maybe I will be a survivor. I don't want to die. I don't think anybody does. But I don't have the paralysing fear that I used to have. I've seen people die with a lot of peace in their faces. Though again I've seen somebody fight for that last breath and not let go.'

John is writing a will to set down what he wants done after he dies. But what John most fears about AIDS isn't dying, but becoming demented before dying.

'I know two people with AIDS dementia and it is very hard to live with. It is hard for them. They don't know who they are or where they are any more. When they are lucid they go through such agony and torment and I would hate that to happen to me. I would rather die of some physical manifestation of AIDS than a neurological one. I would rather die from pneumonia or cancer than lose my grip on reality first and become an non-person even before I am dead.

'But my life now is just so much better than it used to be. I have such high hopes that it is going to get even better. Some people call AIDS "Accelerated Inner Development Syndrome". That is the way I choose to think of it. So I'm looking forward to the challenges of the next few years.'

On 30 October 1988 John Mordaunt got engaged to Andria Efthimiov. John is alive, on AZT, and feeling well. He and Andria are together in London and enjoying life.